OSTEOPATHY
A PATIENT'S GUIDE

by

Edward Triance D.O.

THORSONS PUBLISHING GROUP
Wellingborough * New York

First Published 1986

British Library Cataloguing in Publication Data

Triance, E.R.
  Osteopathy: a patient's guide.
  1.Osteopathy
  I.Title
  615.5'33   RZ341

  ISBN 0-7225-1247-3

Printed and bound in Great Britain

OSTEOPATHY

A Patient's Guide

An introductory guide explaining how osteopathy works and what can be expected when a patient seeks treatment.

Contents

Acknowledgements

My thanks to Howard for his help with the illustrations.

Introduction

Osteopathy has been practised for over 100 years. In the USA, where it was founded, it has very largely become integrated into the main medical system, most osteopaths there are fully trained medical practitioners who have followed their foundation course in colleges with a bias towards osteopathic philosophy. After graduation they may subsequently practise as general practitioners, surgeons, or specialists, and do so alongside those trained in the orthodox establishments, with the advantage of being able to introduce osteopathic treatment when appropriate. The patient may decide whether he/she prefers an osteopathic doctor and has the right to change his/her physician at will.

In the UK osteopathy is practised in a restricted way as an alternative to traditional medicine. Patients seeking osteopathic treatment are not always aware how powerful an alternative therapy it is, its scope extending far beyond the use of manipulative techniques for the treatment of minor physical injuries. Thousands of patients have received osteopathic treatment outside the orthodox medical system, whose practitioners have generally been aware of osteopathic activities but who have chosen to wear medical 'blinkers'.

Fifty years ago many people thought that osteopathy was a treatment using the hands which in some mysterious way healed the sick. During the last twenty years the image of osteopathy has greatly improved. In many ways, however, it has suffered from over exposure of some aspects of its philosophy and treatment, and almost total disregard of others.

Very little factual information is published about its principles and to some extent patients today are more ignorant of them than those seeking treatment fifty years ago. Most publicity given to osteopathy is intermixed with information about other forms of manipulative treatment and portrays osteopaths as 'joint manipulators' with little interest in anything other than 'disc' problems. So much emphasis has been placed upon this classification that patients are very surprised to learn that osteopaths deal with many conditions such as headaches, chest pains and gastric disorders. Most are even more surprised to learn that osteopathic techniques can be used for successfully treating many functional diseases such as insomnia, migraine, vertigo, asthma, enteritis, colitis, ulcers, illness arising from functional disorders affecting the liver, gall bladder or colon, as well as functional cardiac problems. The British patient will find that one osteopath will treat a much broader range of illness than another. In France, however, where the osteopathic profession is very new you will generally find a much more comprehensive approach and practitioners there apply osteopathic principles very widely. These aspects need not worry prospective patients too much as long as they recognize that there are a wide variety of osteopaths who may or may not have the training or experience to deal with their special problems.

In 1892 after thirty-six years of application of its principles its founder Andrew Taylor Still, said 'Osteopathy is in its infancy'. It has since prospered and been enlarged upon by his disciples. A vast amount of material is available at osteopathic research establishments in the USA which both confirms scientifically the principles of osteopathy and records the success of clinical treatment.

It is to be hoped that outside the USA the principles of osteopathy will be integrated into what is now regarded as traditional medicine and that the emerging interest in 'alternative medicine' will form the impetus for a wider acceptance of the importance of mechanical causes of disease and disability.

This book outlines the life of the founder of osteopathy, Andrew Taylor Still, the circumstances which led him to establish an Osteopathic College and his own interpretation of some osteopathic principles. It covers some theory as well as explaining the term osteopathic lesion, a condition central to osteopathic philosophies in the cause of ill health, along with its effects and its treatment. As this book is intended for the patient contemplating osteopathic treatment it gives some indication of what to expect on consultation and the kind of treatments likely to be administered. The treatment of 'disc' injuries for which osteopaths are now renowned is covered and I shall touch briefly upon the subject of cranial osteopathy, a most important area of practice for which only a few practitioners are trained.

History

Chapter 1

History

Andrew Taylor Still was born in Virginia in 1828, the son of a Methodist Minister. As a boy he had some casual experience of caring for the sick as his father ran a Methodist Mission for Indians in Kansas. Initially he trained for five years to become an engineer but subsequently attended the Kansas City School of Physicians and Surgeons around 1855, later becoming an army surgeon involved in the frontier fighting during the Civil War. His medical experiences during the war, combined with the tragic loss of his three children who died during an epidemic of spinal meningitis, caused him to become dispirited with orthodox medical treatment and question its value.

To put the foundation of osteopathy into perspective we must realize what the state of medical practice was in a country as vast as America over 100 years ago. There were virtually no drugs anywhere which had a specific effect on disease, such as iron for the treatment of anaemia or quinine for malaria, and very few drugs had any significant effect in alleviating symptoms. Often these were injected in a haphazard way and the use of leeches, bloodletting and purging with mercury were still common practice. Surgery was then a bloody, brutal business and anaesthetics such as ether and nitrous oxide were modern innovations. What Dr Still felt impelled to do was to find a more compassionate way of dealing with medical problems and also to seek an alternative to the indiscriminate drugging of patients. His early training as an engineer demanded of him that he find logical reasons for the administration of medicinal treatments and his specialized ability to observe and reason led to an honest disappointment with the practice of medicine. Haphazard prescriptions gave no reasonable grounds on which to forecast results accurately and his observations of the physician's failure to help the sick in seemingly simple and uncomplicated cases with the best medical care available led him to renounce the use of drugs.

Had he lived today he might not have felt so passionately about disposing of every drug. But preparations such as insulin for diabetes or erlichs salvarsan for syphilis had not been discovered then and it is easy to appreciate the reasons for his search for an alternative method. The standard method of treatment for pneumonia, for example, included applying hot bags, administering morphine, whisky, digitalis or strychnine. He discovered that manual methods alone were remarkably more effective in a very high percentage of cases.

In 1874 he began to use manual techniques, which he called osteopathy, in conjunction with surgery and built up a very big practice, becoming renowned over a wide area for the good results he achieved. Eighteen years later, having proved that these techniques were infinitely more effective than available treatment, he founded the first School of Osteopathic Medicine in Kirksville, Missouri. Osteopathic schools have since developed and flourished alongside the schools of orthodox medicine and taught 'improved systems of surgery, obstetrics and treatment of disease generally'. The graduates of these schools were to be competent in all medical matters, but used osteopathic techniques whenever possible in preference to any other treatment because they were trained with an osteopathic approach. It is important to realize that Dr Still did not dismiss every medical theory but sought a new approach to the treatment of disease with an emphasis on mechanical causes. His friend and colleague in the establishment of the first school was a surgeon from Edinburgh who, like him, believed it was necessary to perform operations both for the repair and for the correction of conditions which prevented normal function of the body in ill health. He would not, however, have performed an operation such as the removal of tonsils unless convinced that it was absolutely necessary and that their condition was not merely a manifestation of an expression of ill health in the whole individual.

In the USA the modern osteopath receives full medical training and there are osteopathic physicians as well as osteopathic surgeons. Today there are seven osteopathic colleges, hundreds of osteopathic hospitals and thousands of osteopathic physicians. Many osteopathic physicians are general practitioners and, although they have the same scope of medical practice as orthodox doctors of medicine, they emphasize the importance of normal body mechanics and the philosophies of Dr Still in their diagnosis and treatment.

Outside the USA osteopaths do not have the same medical status and some colleges have survived in spite of the dominance of the long-established medical schools. If it were not for the Common Law, which is unique in the United Kingdom, it is unlikely that the development of osteopathy could have progressed before the 1940s. Its practice in the countries of the EEC was illegal until relatively recently. Although osteopaths outside the USA train for a long period and are required to uphold high standards of entrance and qualification, their colleges are small and do not have access to full medical training facilities. Only those practitioners who become fully qualified osteopaths after having qualified as physicians or surgeons have similar status to their counterparts in the USA. In consequence, osteopaths are restricted to private practice and work entirely on their own. They are inevitably limited in some potential areas of their work but can still provide very effective help in a wide range of illnesses. That they have survived and distinguished themselves by bringing relief to millions of patients is evidence of the truth of a great part of Dr Still's theory.

Chapter 2

Some Theory

The alternative approach which Dr Still followed when he founded the first osteopathic school was, no doubt, influenced by his early training as an engineer. He frequently presented his theories in engineering terms, with constant analogy to the newly invented steam engine. Much of what he wrote was often ridiculed outside America, and his writings are still inclined to be misquoted when taken out of context, but his intuition and intellect led him to make assessments, the scientific aspects of which are still being demonstrated.

He recognized nature's role in health and disease, stating that a good physician should know how to assist nature in maintaining or building the *homeo-static* forces that lead to health. Here are three basic principles which he emphasized and which are still valid today:

1. The normal healthy body contains within itself the mechanism of defence and repair in injuries resulting from trauma, infections and other toxic agents.
2. The body is a unit, and abnormal structure or function in one part exerts abnormal influence on other parts.
3. The body can function best in defence or repair when it has maximum structural mobility and flexibility.

That the body has built-in defences against disease is now, of course, an indisputable fact. We now know, for instance, that scientific studies of the lymphatic system have confirmed its function as a defence against infection, and that resistance is the natural reaction of healthy living cells to invading germs or

microbes, which only become virulent when they find a
vulnerably sub-vital and morbid state of the blood and tissues in
which they can breed.

Dr Still taught his pupils that the body makes its own life-
giving, life-preserving and healing substances. Today we would
call this concept *biological*. Perhaps we should look at Dr Still's
own words on this subject:

> ... that all remedies necessary to health exist in the human body in
> such condition that the remedies may naturally associate
> themselves together and relieve the afflicted.

The corollary to the idea of the body having its own defence
mechanism was that as a general rule illness developed when
the defences were weakened and that such weakness was
brought about, among other things, by the body going
mechanically wrong.

When confronted with illness, Dr Still 'stood back', as it
were, and viewed the *whole* patient. He abandoned the usual
medical practice of treating the symptoms without satisfying
himself about the causes.

Inevitably, in considering the whole person and investigating
all his/her problems, he started from an evaluation of the basic
structure, namely the skeleton. He took everyting into
consideration — height, weight, posture, age, deportment and
locomotion, deformities whether congenital, developed or as a
result of accident, the range of movement of every joint. From
there he examined the muscles and ligaments which held the
skeleton together — their length, tone, general condition, any
evidence of wastage, any spasticity or flaccidity. He was deeply
concerned both with the action of the muscles as operating
levers of the body and with their performance in the support of
the joints.

Next, his examination would include the connective tissues
which he would locate wherever possible by deep and gentle
searching with his fingers. This examination would include
what is called the *fascia*. The fascia consists of bands or sheets of

fibro-elastic tissue which envelopes the whole body beneath the surface of the skin. It forms many sheaths to enclose muscles as well as organs and nerves. Special consideration would be given to some areas such as the neck where stresses on certain fascia can easily be located. During his examination Dr Still would most likely have examined manually the internal organs, such as the stomach and liver, in much the same way as the old-fashioned medical doctor searching for clues to illness throughout the entire body but identifying physical problems. Dr Still emphasized the importance of thorough examination:

> I want the attention of the engineer because to him a fact is a truth. He reasons with ability. He always halts at the diseased points either of muscle or bone. He makes his conclusion as to the cause that has produced the abnormal condition from the cause of friction which has produced adhesion of bone, disease of bone, inflammation and disease of flesh or whatever be the abnormality...

and on another occasion he said:

> ... this subject is too serious not to come under the most crucial and exact requirements of which human skill is master. If a mechanic is so particular to inspect *every part* and principle belonging to a steam engine for the purpose of getting good results, can you as an engineer omit any bone in the body and claim to be a trustworthy engineer? Can you say that *any part* has no importance physiologically in the engine of life. Remember your responsibility in the sick room. You must reason or fail.

This kind of approach is what today we label *holistic*.

Dr Still's concept of the body's resistance to ailments taught him to search for the actual condition that produced the symptoms. Every doctor is, of course, concerned with the signs of disease and symptoms but the osteopath is most concerned with causes, often quite remote from the site of the malady.

Dr Still believed that many causes of illness, as well as the factors which led to them, could be found chiefly in the structure of the body. By *structure* he meant the whole body, the skeleton, the muscles, the fascia, the organs and even the skin. He did not ever state, as he is often misrepresented as doing, that all illness is caused by disorder of the joints of the spine. He never even said that *all* illness was caused by disorder of the structure. What he did teach was that *structure* and *function* are inextricably interrelated. These are his words:

> The body's musculoskeletal system, the bones, the ligaments, the muscles, the fascia, form a structure which when disordered can effect changes in the function of other parts of the body.

You will see later how this important subject affects you as a patient.

Contrary to generally accepted ideas held today, Dr Still placed as much significance in diagnosis and treatment on the fascia as the spine. This was his advice:

> The fascia is the place to look for the cause of the disease and the place to consult and begin the action of remedies in all diseases.

This insistence on the importance of the fascia cannot be overstated, and Dr Still wrote at great length much that has since been verified by modern research.

These ideas of structure and function and the importance of the fascia, together with other important concepts enunciated by Dr Still are introduced more fully later. Meanwhile, I shall discuss the areas of structure outlined above and explain what a modern osteopath does before arriving at a diagnosis or giving any treatment. This will enable you to know what kind of examination to expect and the reasons for it.

Chapter 3

Osteopathic Examination

An osteopath will first examine the problem area and then turn his attention to the superstructure of the body — the skeleton. As our skeleton, unlike that of insects and invertebrates, is inside our bodies and does not form its protective shell, we cannot see the actual condition of it. An osteopath, however, is trained to examine a patient in a way which will give him a very considerable amount of information about a patient's general health, occupation and even life history by pure observation. Before he even lays a finger on a patient an experienced osteopath will have noted the way the patient walked into the consulting room, the way the body is held in posture, and the amount of mobility and control when asked to sit down. The way a patient carried his/her head, for example, can give immediate clues as to the condition of the curves of the spine and often on disorders as far removed from the carriage of the head as the difference in leg length.

When a patient is undressed the trained eye of the osteopath will immediately recognize a host of structural conditions which may influence the state of health. Examination of a patient sitting, standing or lying down will show the general overall balance of the body. A mental note will be made of such characteristics as a short leg, a tilted pelvis, a lowered shoulder, inequality of the height of shoulder blades, overexaggerated curves of the spine (kyphosis), unnatural curvature (scoliosis), round shoulders, forward carriage of the neck and head, unusual development of the legs and feet and so forth — all of which might *induce* physical illness. The osteopath then makes tests to check not only the efficiency of movement of the main joints of the body but also every spinal joint.

Dr Still said that *motion* was the connection between structure and function. The consideration of motion at this stage in the osteopathic examination is of prime importance. When an osteopath examines his patient he is not likely, for instance, to overlook the movement of the rib cage or its significance in relation to the patient's breathing. So he is concerned with movement — in the range of the joints, in the spinal segments, in the rib cage and indeed, the full range of movement of the whole body. More significantly he is concerned with restriction of movement, or *motion discordance*.

The Skeleton

Before continuing any further it should be emphasized that no human being is a perfectly formed structure. Many basic structural patterns are, of course, inherited but, quite naturally, or perhaps unnaturally, a person's mode of life affects their posture. The variations of postural change resulting from occupation are innumerable.

Clearly if a person spends 50 per cent of his/her life standing over a machine, typing letters, writing up accounts, watching a VDU screen or pulling levers, to name a few examples, then consequential changes of posture must take place and after a while the shape of the skeleton will change, particularly in the way it fits together and in the way it *moves*. The osteopath will relate his findings not merely to the problem with which the patient has presented him but also to the factors that led to the problem arising. We shall subsequently see the need for this when we have considered the other parts of the structure and their relevance to treatment.

We should mention here that although skeletal formation is of extreme importance in osteopathic diagnosis this examination is not carried out in order to ascertain what should be done to alter it. It is not osteopathic intention to 'straighten out' the basic structure of a patient. Any idea that the basic structure of a patient could be altered directly by manipulative treatment would be quite ludicrous. Just as a gardener knows that it is not possible to straighten out the stem of a plant that has grown distorted, so it is that an osteopath appreciates that the spine cannot be 'straightened' but, like a gardener, he will know that it may sometimes be retrained into better shape. Success in retraining would naturally be more probable in a young patient. The spine is a living structure of which the cells are undergoing reconstruction and it obviously forms in the pattern of its environment. The structural features of modern man will have a direct relationship with his life and occupation in civilized society.

Dr Still described bone as 'a laboratory'. Many people assume that the bones of the human skeleton are solid, stable and immutable, which is the impresssion that you get if you study a model skeleton. This is totally misleading. Bone is, in fact, a living tissue which has blood vessels and nerves of its own and it is influenced by all the factors that influence any of the softer structures of the body.

Bone is moulded by its environment and can change in response to stresses and strains and it is therefore, essentially plastic in nature. The inorganic basis of bone, which forms 60 per cent of it, is undergoing continual renewal during a person's life. You will gather from this, then, that a skeleton can be trained to alter its shape by altering its environment over a long period of time; that it is certainly possible to train the growth of a skeleton by controlling postural habits during the formative years of growing up; that if a skeleton suffers a major injury such as a broken femur which results in the shortening of a leg, for example, the consequent imbalance will, in the course of time, throw the structure out of line and cause stresses that will eventually alter the shape and surfaces of the joints and even the shape of the bones themselves. The effects of such injury on the symmetry of the structure would be much greater if it happened during childhood. This is an example of the relationship between *function* and *structure*.

The Muscles

Of initial interest to the osteopath will be those muscles which are concerned with the posture of the patient. If the osteopath observed that there were problems with the skeleton then the muscles which supported the affected structure would be specially examined. If, for example, there was a forward curvature of the spine (lordosis) the large muscles supporting the spine would be examined, first separately, and then in relation to the whole posture. The osteopath's concern is not to compare any patient with a skeletal blueprint, but to assess what is normal for that patient — 'No two persons are alike'. The osteopath sees what is, in fact, the results of the efforts of that patient's structure to attain or maintain a symmetry in the face of the *functional* demands which have been made upon it during its lifetime. Osteopathy does not regard peculiarities of structure as strictly 'abnormal'. It assesses how the patient's structure has *adapted* to the life it has led.

Unless the posture has changed from what is usually normal for the patient because of recent injury, such as a prolapsed disc, osteopathy does not advocate that it should be corrected by any direct treatment. If treatment were necessary in such circumstances it would be a very gradual programme and involve, as your may realize, corrective exercises.

The muscles involved in the support and control of any joints that are not functioning properly will be carefully examined. Those that have been concerned in recent injury will receive immediate attention.

The Surface

After examining the muscles the osteopath will carry out careful examination of the surface of the body using a very specialized technique generally known as 'palpation'. Palpation is the chief art of the skilful osteopath and enables him to detect structural changes, sometimes quite minute, which might have very radical effects over a wide area and affect the working of the structures in other parts of the body which are supplied through connecting nerve pathways. His hands are his chief diagnostic instrument and the quality of an osteopath and the depth of his training can be judged by his ability here. An experienced practitioner will rapidly locate causes of physical complaints after light palpation in suspected areas. With deeper palpation he will trace origins of a vast range of problems. Disorders which will concern him are tenderness, hardened or 'ropy' muscle, fibrotic changes, signs of immobility in the muscles and connective tissues themselves, the state of the muscle 'tone' and areas of inflammation or minor swelling. Not least he will find out the condition of supporting ligaments and tendons and changes in the relationship of joints. This examination will cause the patient no discomfort at all and palpation does not involve digging fingers into the tissues or performing friction-type movements.

The Fascia

Deeper palpation is, of course, necessary for examination of the fascia. A good osteopath will make a very thorough examination of all connective tissues. Again he will be searching for a very wide range of possible causes of illness. Not merely will he be appraising the tissues in their role as supporting structures but he will be studying their relationship and the effects of strain upon such important matters as breathing. He will look for evidence of inflammation and trace concentrations of collagenous fibres. The secondary effects of fascial strain produce compression, swelling and stretching of nerve trunks. These in turn bring about pain or interference with nerve impulses, blood, or lymph supply to local areas as you will see later. Those areas which the medical profession describe as 'trigger spots' will be included in this examination. The more specific problems of the patient's illness will naturally receive special consideration but not in an isolated way. Each practitioner will proceed in a different way and add a variety of diagnostic procedures which he feels are applicable to the individual case. One thing he will do is assure himself that the patient cannot in any way be harmed by the treatment he is proposing.

Although the process may sound 'over thorough' and perhaps arduous for the patient you will find that an experienced osteopath will not take an unreasonable time over it and, in fact, osteopathic diagnosis can often be made quite quickly.

Osteopathic examination differs from that of current medical practice, which is more concerned with the identification of specific diseases than with non-specific conditions that exist before specific diseases arise. The osteopathic approach to examination, then, is essentially of a *biological* and *holistic* nature.

Chapter 4

Osteopathic Lesions

We shall now consider in more detail the theoretical and practical matters which the osteopath is trained to apply in his appraisal of the patient, and their relevance to the diagnosis.

We shall briefly study the condition which has brought osteopathy most success, helped it to gain public respect and, during the last few years, initiated a change in the attitude of the general medical profession. We are referring to a condition which is often termed 'back trouble'. Because of their outstanding success in the treatment of back complaints many people have grown to regard osteopaths as practitioners who simply treat backs. This they undoubtedly are and will continue to succeed to be since it is inevitable that any practitioner trained to search for the causes of ill health by meticulous examination of the structure should know considerably more about its working mechanics than any other therapist. Treatment for back complaints, however, is only a very small part of the scope of osteopathic therapeutics.

Osteopathic diagnosis includes a particular condition that may occur in *any joint* which is usually described as the 'osteopathic lesion'. This was not, incidentally, a term used by Dr Still who preferred 'derangement', but because much misunderstanding existed about what osteopaths were doing to achieve successful results, without what medical establishments considered to be scientific explanation, it was felt necessary to find a scientific base to describe the condition they treated. 'Osteopathic lesion' was the outcome and you will hear osteopaths referring to lesions when explaining their diagnosis.

Nearly seventy years of research has been made into their causes, existence and effects, and volumes of factual information are available, especially in the USA. The word lesion which is derived from the Latin *laesio* is, of course, used by the medical profession to describe an injury or wound, and it was not common for doctors to talk of lesions of the spine unless they meant quite serious injury. However, as their interest in osteopathy grows they are becoming acquainted with the different use of the term.

Every joint of the human body is designed to move through a certain *limited range*. For our purposes here we shall describe the movement of joints of any individual as *normal* where there has been no cogenital deformity or severe injury which might have damaged, changed or prevented the free movement of joints, or any illness or disease which has caused pathological conditions to alter the movement of joints.

Joints are supported by ligaments, tendons and muscles, as well as the fascia, and are bound together by sheaths. These either permit or bring about the movement of joints of each individual within a *limited range special* to that person. Some people have a wider range of movement in their joints than others for many different reasons.

When there is a shift of a joint, in any direction, in a way that is not usual for the design of that joint than sometimes a jam or fixation occurs. The joint is then *held* by the supporting ligaments, tendons, muscles and sheaths in a position which is the *extreme limit of its normal range*.

When the joint continues to be held in this position of extreme limit we have a situation which osteopaths describe as an osteopathic lesion. You will notice that I have very carefully emphasized that the joint is jammed in a position at the extreme limit of its *normal* range because if it were jammed in a position beyond its normal range it would not be an osteopathic lesion but a dislocation or partial dislocation. Because joints are jammed in positions at the limit of their normal range any X-rays may not be likely to show anything that a non-osteopathic practitioner would consider to be of orthopaedic importance.

This is why much frustration is expressed by patients, who having been told that X-rays are 'clear' by their GP have sought osteopathic help and obtained relief. Patients having experienced movement of joints which apparently brought relief of symptoms during osteopathic treatment cannot understand why the trouble was not diagnosed earlier, especially if X-rays have been taken.

The osteopathic lesion therefore, is not a very great movement of bones but more a slight yielding of the joint and a fixing of it at the limit of its normal range of movement.

Osteopaths do deal with other forms of disorganization of the joints but that part of their work is outside this present discussion. Osteopathic lesions are of such great importance that they need to be understood by everyone seeking osteopathic help. An osteopathic lesion must be accurately diagnosed before any treatment can be contemplated. Treatment given by an inexperienced practitioner in a random way may seem to help symptoms but may very well be harmful later or at best only give temporary relief, especially if no regard in diagnosis has been shown for the factors which induced the problems. As accurate diagnosis is so vital training in this skill is involved and lengthy. Mechancial tests are used to establish what is the normal range of movement of the individual patient. These are followed by tests to locate the joints which are restricted, combined with further diagnostic techniques using palpation.

Chapter 5

The Effects of Osteopathic Lesions

Before I attempt to identify some of the damaging effects of an osteopathic lesion, I must re-emphasize that it occurs in *any joint* of the body and that it is bound up with *total body mechanics*. As we shall see, the effects of an osteopathic lesion can appear to be out of all proportion to a cause which is no more than a minor fixation of a joint within its normal range. However, if the moment that the yielding of the joint occurred is studied in the light of all the postural and mechanical factors which induced it to happen, it will be seen more as part of a *process* which will continue if not reversed. Osteopathic treatment cannot be conveniently reduced to the neat idea that 'one bone out of position causes symptoms which are automatically remedied when that bone is put back into position'. A patient should try to abandon this concept completely and think in terms of *total* structural appraisal. Even if acute symptoms which brought a patient to an osteopath are relieved, the causative factors will remain unless something is done to alter or arrest them.

To simplify the idea of cause and effect consider the following practical experiments. Look at a very small vein in the back of your hand and apply pressure to it with the thumb of your other hand for, say, 25 seconds. You will notice when you take your thumb off how long it takes for the blood to return to the compressed area. Should you keep the pressure up for, say, 60 seconds you may begin to experience a slight numbing sensation and after 100 seconds begin to sense what you might recognise as minor pain. Should you want a more dramatic demonstration put a tight elastic band around your index finger and see how quickly you experience the sensation of numbness, fullness and gradually increasing discomfort.

Most people have known the frustration of not being able to start their car and been relieved to find that by merely removing a terminal attached to the battery and wiping it lightly before reconnecting it their car started instantly. All motor breakdown specialists know how a screw in the middle of a distributor can loosen very slightly and result in disorder of the running or even complete breakdown of the car. Similarly, health is a matter of perfect equilibrium and its balance may be disturbed by seemingly trifling circumstances. You may reason that the domestic difficulties we have mentioned arise from lack of care or regular servicing and this is a matter we shall examine with regard to the body later. What we are observing is the operation of a law formulated by Maupertius, a French mathematician; namely, that the quantity of action necessary to effect any change in nature is the least possible. Osteopathically speaking, the amount of derangement from normal mobility needed to start a process of ill health with marked clinical reaction is very small.

Let us apply this idea to just three or four parts of the anatomy where an osteopathic lesion can occur. First, visualize a bone, or vertebra, in the spine. Each spinal joint has a small opening (foramen) through which pass the root nerves from the spinal cord itself. The space is only big enough to allow the passage of a nerve fibre and is packed with tissue and bathed in fluid. There is no room for any great movement of the fibre beyond the usual amount which occurs in everyday action of the body. Imagine what happens if there is a very slight yielding of the joint between that bone and the one below and then the joints become fixed or jammed. Remember that the spinal bones are supported and operated by innumerable muscles, sheaths and fascia, that the whole spine must have an unrestricted and flexible sway and is affected by almost *every movement* of the body, and that these muscles and fascia actually lift the trunk and hold it steady.

Lower Back

If this bone we are referring to were to be, say, in the lower back it would be easy to see the detrimental effects of such a restriction. Each time movement occurs beyond a certain range the muscles and fascia will be hurt or strained to a varying degree and a sudden jerky movement beyond that range could cause them to be sprained, sometimes severely. Alternatively if there was no accident of that sort but a person with an osteopathic lesion felt only minor discomfort and stiffness and their everyday activities were unaffected unless they made certain specific movements, they might 'live with' the condition avoiding things which aggravated it. What then? Then we have a local area affected by the stress which this restriction produces. When I say stress I mean resistance of the body to strain which is necessary to allow *motion*. The parts affected may become inflamed, tender or even swollen. The circulation of the blood in the tiny nearby capillaries is restricted and may be shut off. This blood is the means of providing nutrition to the joint. Without going deeply into the importance of free circulation it is easy to appreciate that a similar condition will be found in this small area surrounding the joint as arises when an elastic band is tightened around an index finger. Any area of the body deprived of proper nerve or blood supply, and consequently nutrition, will eventually become diseased.

Trapped Nerves

One of the most common effects of an osteopathic lesion is the entrapment of nerves. This is an idea that almost everybody now seems to grasp and frequently patients say that they think they have a 'nerve trapped' before any consultation takes place. Frequently it is suggested that nerves are trapped by discs in the spine. This can in a way be true but is, in fact, not the commonest occurrence.

A human has thirty one pairs of nerves which originate in the spinal cord and these pass through the fibrous tunnels or apertures (foramen) in the bones of the spine (the vertebrae) we have mentioned. These are described as roots and are the origins of a two-way nerve pathway which, on the one hand, supplies the muscles of the body as well as the organs with power to function and, on the other, receives information from the whole structure which is in turn transmitted back to the brain. (This is, of course, a gross oversimplification of a complicated subject in which osteopaths must of necessity have thorough training.)

The divisions of nerve fibres are arranged in groups each called a plexus which supply different areas of the body.

Brachial Plexus

Let us take as an example of a plexus the Brachial Plexus, which arises in the upper back and supplies all the muscles of the arm (see Figure 1). An osteopathic lesion in a joint of the spine where this plexus emanates could cause mechanical irritation of one of the root nerves passing through the aperture (foramen) and so *directly* bring about pain, loss of sensation and loss of power to any part of the arm as far away as the fingers, or it might cause the symptoms to occur more locally in the area of the shoulder blade, or sometimes both. Anything which causes increased pressure on the roots, such as a stretching action or a cough, will increase pain. Early diagnosis and release of an osteopathic lesion will very quickly relieve these particular symptoms. Because an osteopathic lesion immobilizes the joint, and the muscles, tendons and fascia are trying to move a joint which is restricted, it will in turn cause strain on those muscles, tendons and fascia. This will again result in inflammation of the structures involved. Whenever muscles, tendons and fascia pass over nerves there is always a possibility of trapping them there, especially at places where the nerve fibres change their course across fibrous bands.

Since osteopathic lesions can occur in *any* joint of the body you will realize that any restriction of the shoulder, elbow, wrist or any joints of the arm or hand will result in the same problems arising, particulary below the level of the joint concerned. In that way some part of the nerve fibres which are supplied from the brachial plexus will be trapped either near to the joint or at

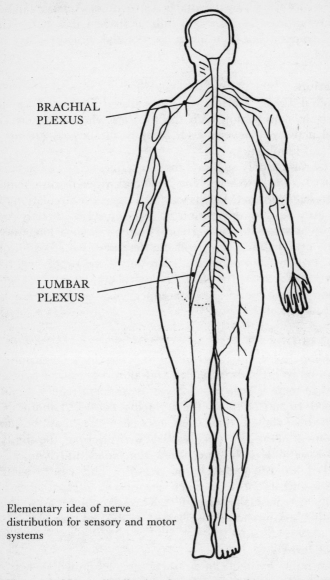

BRACHIAL
PLEXUS

LUMBAR
PLEXUS

Elementary idea of nerve
distribution for sensory and motor
systems

Figure 1.   Nerve distribution for sensory and motor systems.

some distance from it by the attached structures. A nerve can be indirectly affected and become inflamed when it is not itself actually trapped but is near to part of the structure that is restricted.

Circulation

The spinal bones (vertebrae) are encased in fascia which contracts in conjunction with the muscles whenever there is physical activity. Between each layer of fascia pass arteries, nerves and lymphatics.

The fascia not only supports these arteries, veins and nerves etc., but also works to keep veins open and widen or close them when muscles contract. In this way they assist the circulation of blood. Any spasm or tension in the muscles, directly or indirectly attached to the vertebral column even a long way from the osteopathic lesion, will interfere with the freedom of the fascia to do this work and, as a result, blood supply will be restricted and may be cut off. Pathological conditions can then arise and may have serious consequences if the condition is allowed to persist.

Damage to Disc

If an osteopathic lesion is permitted to persist for a long time it becomes more difficult to relieve and after a period of two or three years there is little possibility of permanent relief without prolonged re-education of the inducing causes. Laboratory research has shown that even though there may be no displacement of the disc lying between the vertebrae, the ability of that disc to absorb water from the blood and lymph is reduced if an osteopathic lesion persists. This causes some shrinkage and its job as a shock absorber is affected since it gradually loses its cushioning effect. This is another reason why osteopathic lesions should be released as soon as possible.

Wear of Joint

The continuing existence of an osteopathic lesion will increase the probability of wear on any joint for the very same reason that a moving part of any structure or machinery which is regulary placed under stress will be much more susceptible to wear and strain when it is out of alignment.

Nerve Pathways

Most of us have become familiar with the use of home computers and, in order to explain its behaviour, the function of the brain has been likened to a computer. It would, perhaps, be more appropriate to say that the spinal cord is like a computer and the brain more like the person operating it. The root nerves relate to the interfaces between the various parts of equipment in the very sophisticated systems of the body. Scientists have not identified to any conclusive degree connections between parts of the brain and individual actions of the body, with the partial exception of the hindbrain (cerebellum). Once the forebrain (cerebrum) has learned any new movements which require concentration, such as walking, swimming, dancing or cycling, it hands the controls over to the hindbrain (cerebellum) which harmonizes all movements and works in an unconscious way in conjunction with the spinal cord. The hindbrain is, as it were, programmed to deal with learned activities. This is not exactly true, of course, but will be a useful analogy to explain nerve pathways. As the nerve pathways are a two-way system we will have to assume that the hindbrain and the spinal cord are programmed to deliver instructions and to act upon information received from the sensory impulses (see Figure 2). If we think of nerve pathways in terms of patterns similar to those seen as graphics on a screen and the same patterns as an extension of those running through the hindbrain and spinal cord you will grasp the idea that they do not work in a fragmented way but as a broad pattern. When the lines of nerve patterns reach the various vertebrae they separate out to serve different parts of the body, the muscles and organs etc., in the form of tiny fibres. When there is a mistake in a program you experience some distortion of graphics on your screen and, likewise, when the wrong information is received by the brain and the spinal cord, your

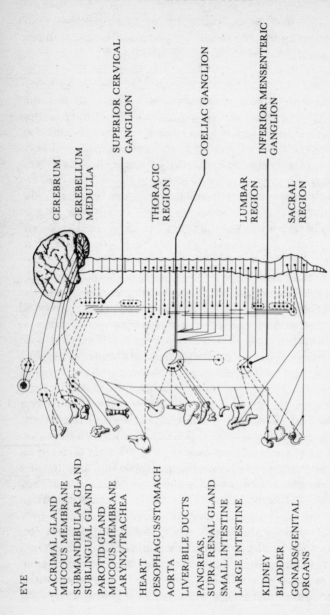

EYE

LACRIMAL GLAND
MUCOUS MEMBRANE
SUBMANDIBULAR GLAND
SUBLINGUAL GLAND
PAROTID GLAND
MUCOUS MEMBRANE
LARYNX/TRACHEA

HEART

OESOPHAGUS/STOMACH
AORTA
LIVER/BILE DUCTS
PANCREAS,
SUPRA RENAL GLAND
SMALL INTESTINE
LARGE INTESTINE

KIDNEY
BLADDER
GONADS/GENITAL
ORGANS

CEREBRUM
CEREBELLUM
MEDULLA
SUPERIOR CERVICAL
GANGLION

THORACIC
REGION

COELIAC GANGLION

LUMBAR
REGION

SACRAL
REGION

INFERIOR MENSENTERIC
GANGLION

The illustration shows how the organs of the body are supplied by *two* sets of nerve fibres. One from the midbrain, medulla and sacral region and another relayed from the thoracic and lumbar regions from large ganglia lying near to the spinal column.

Figure 2. The organs of the body are served by two sets of nerve fibres.

human computer will display distorted graphics. When there is a disorganization of the vertebrae which enclose the nerve fibres there arises interference with both input and output. Incorrect information may be received by and issued from the cerebellum and spinal cord. Anyone who has attempted to walk on a leg when experiencing pins and needles will know the sensation and difficulties of co-ordination that occur when the brain is receiving wrong information. Continued interference can be detrimental to the local area of the spinal cord. Bearing in mind that these signals (impulses) are also responsible for the functioning of the visceral organs of the body, it is logical to conclude that a vertebral disorganization can in some way be detrimental to the health of those organs. Disturbance at any position along a nerve fibre can arise as a result of an osteopathic lesion in any part of the structure adjacent to it, a wrist, elbow, shoulder etc., or where the fascia may have become swollen or formed an adhesion. These disturbances are greatest where fibres pass across bones, and especially at the roots in the spinal area. Nerve impulses are conducted in a rhythmical way and compression of a nerve fibre will create a disruption of that rhythm and excite the impulse. The functions which those nerve fibres bring about may not be wholly cut off; they may not even be very obviously disturbed or handicapped but the patterns will be distorted and insidious symptoms arise. Every instruction that the brain gives involves an extraordinary number of patterns because each movement we make is incredibly complicated; so it is more accurate to think of disturbed patterns to and from the spinal cord than to think of one nerve fibre being compressed and one signal or impulse being disturbed.

Osteopaths, excluding some in the USA, are not scientists and clearly do not have neurological expertise, nor can they with any degree of accuracy trace the exact origins of disturbance of nerve supply to any sick organ of the body. What they know from actual experience is that constitutional symptoms very frequently diminish and disappear after osteopathic lesions are released and that proven patterns of

disorder can be related to specific joints of the spine. The
occurrence of this phenomenon has been recorded for over 100
years and is too regularly seen to dismiss as co-incidental. What
they can do is ensure that all osteopathic lesions are located and
relieved before constitutional symptoms begin to develop. Dr
Still advised, 'If there are any bony variations, if muscles or
nerves are oppressed remove the cause and the result is *harmony*
and it is felt throughout the system'.

Chemico therapy in such conditions may be effective to
alleviate the symptoms but cannot remove them and must
perforce be continued if the causes are not eradicated. Once
organic disease has become established, however, permanent
damage of the organs will eventually result and osteopathic
treatment would become ineffective in relieving it.

The Hip Joint

Let us turn our attention very briefly to another part of the
structure of the body which may be subject to an osteopathic
lesion: the hip joint (see Figure 3). This has an important
function in supporting the pelvis which is a bridge upon which
the superstructure of the body must balance. A yielding and
fixing of this joint at the limit of its normal range may for
simplicity be described as a hip shift. Even a minor shift of the
hip will cause extreme pain down the front of the thigh and into
the groin as well as marked disability when walking. Dr Still
identified disorganization of the hip as the cause of the
development of a wide variety of disease-producing conditions.
Because the hip joint is very large the consequences of its
restriction are much more obvious. Often, however, a patient
suffering from quite severe symptoms may not, in fact, realize
that the hip itself is restricted. The ligaments and muscles of the
pelvis bind the hip to form an even brace which must maintain
equilibrium when resisting weight of the trunk which it carries.
Any deviation of the hip from its normal position will cause the
bracing effect to be partially lost. This will result in the weight
of the trunk forcing the sacro-iliac joint to spread. The sacro
-iliac joints are then in danger of giving way under extra strain.

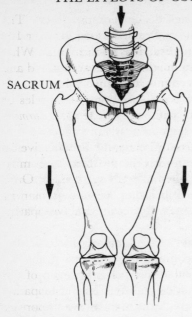

SACRUM

The hip joints support the pelvis in the same way as stanchions support a bridge. Forward displacement of the hip will cause the sacral joints to jam under the downward stress of the structures above.

The sacral joints are covered by a complex mass of vital nerves embedded in fascia, muscles and tendons.

SACRO-ILIAC JOINT

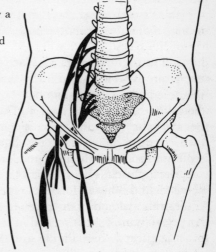

Figure 3.   The hip joints support the pelvis.

The muscles and ligaments on one side, or perhaps both, will in turn cause compression upon the nerves and blood vessels, not least on the femoral and sciatic nerves. The result of this can be pain in the sacro-iliac area, pain down the whole length of the leg, perhaps as far as the big toe, some loss of feeling, pins and needles and burning sensations.

When the patient with a hip shift walks or sits, the strain across the brace of the pelvis will cause a twisting effect on the large pelvic bones. This will usually strain the lumbar bones which are carried above together with the muscles, ligaments and fascia supporting them and often affect posture as far away as the base of the skull. If the hip is not released from this restriction other osteopathic lesions will later inevitably occur in the joints of the lumbar spine.

Compression of the root nerves of the lumbar vertebrae will automatically result and such conditions as sciatica probably follow. Since nerves from the lumbar and pelvic area supply all the vital organs of the lower abdomen, such as the bladder, uterus and part of the colon, the patterns of the nerve pathways to these organs will in turn be distorted.

Inside the pelvis a complicated structure comprising thirty six muscles will suffer from tension, especially on the side that the hip is shifted and effects will spread after continuous motion as the patient performs everyday activities. The pelvis is also full of tendons, ligaments and fascia through which nerves pass and which support the abdominal organs and assist with their operation, blood supply and nutrition. The tension created by the twisting effect of the pelvic bones will logically be transferred to these tendons, ligaments and fascia and so unnaturally strain them, compressing the nerves and blood vessels involved. The resulting disharmony and detrimental effects should be easy to envisage.

The only method of drainage of the organs contained within the pelvis is through the abdominal veins. Any tension that might impede the circulation and drainage can readily be seen to induce such conditions as congestion of the bladder, weakening of the pelvic floor or, in the case of women, torsion of the ligamentous system from which the uterus is suspended. Should such physical disturbances be allowed to continue, symptoms of disease may very well develop.

The muscles of the hip are attached to it in such a way as to pull the hip joint into the socket when they are functioning normally. If, however, a shift has occurred the pelvis will be tipped forward and the hip will loose its stability. A patient with this condition will have difficulty in walking and continued irritation of the joint will cause arthritis.

Other Joints
Let us briefly consider how often very minor restrictions in the movement of joints such as the shoulder, the knee, the ankle, or even a rib may bring about problems in the spine and produce osteopathic lesions there.

To illustrate this idea let us look at the ankle. The structure of the ankle joint combined with that of the lower leg is designed to absorb the shocks from the big thigh bones above. The weight of the body above is distributed evenly through the foot and control is exercised by the muscles and ligaments supporting the ankle. A very common minor injury occurs when there is a turning of the ankle. This commonly happens during sustained repetitive action such as running, an example being when a runner puts one foot into a small divot or strikes uneven ground and the foot is suddenly turned under. This causes strain on the ankle joint which may bring pain or swelling with discomfort lasting a few days or sometimes discomfort alone which tends to persist. Occasionally the ankle may be sprained, but what is more common is a simple shift of the joint within its normal range of movement. Standard orthopaedic examination will not reveal anything of clinical importance and rest is usually recommended. Some discomfort or perhaps swelling continues for a long time and is aggravated by running and sometimes walking. Physiotherapy may help to alleviate the symptoms in the early stages, especially if there is swelling. It is common when acute symptoms subside for the sufferer to endure stoically the residual discomfort which is at its worst during or after activity. During prolonged activity the sufferer will instinctively protect the ankle by transferring some weight to the other foot and thereby create an imbalance in weight distribution. This will gradually bring about changes in balance throughout the entire body even as high as the top of the neck. If the condition is allowed to persist for a long time permanent shortening of the ligaments may take place in the leg, in the pelvis, and particularly in the back and in the neck. These subtle changes will gradually cause other osteopathic lesions to occur in the related spinal areas. At first these may cause only minor discomfort but the muscles which endeavour to maintain balance while undergoing strain may develop a generalized fibrosis, leading to fibrositis. Over a period of many years disturbance of the harmony of walking may result in anatomic changes in the muscles, ligaments and fascia. Any further minor accidents such as a back strain will be likely to result in other osteopathic lesions.

Children

Osteopathic lesions experienced by children are more often than not ignored and treated as growing pains. The small, but accumulating, disturbances of balance will make the individual much more vulnerable to other restrictions of joints even though they may only cause occasional discomfort from postural strain during the formative years. However, organic disturbances may manifest themselves in later life.

Stress Symptoms

Many patients with osteopathic lesions develop fatigue, irritability and vague symptoms which do not fit medical diagnosis. Sometimes they are considered to be neurotic. Correction of osteopathic lesions relieve the undiagnosable symptoms which have drained their energy and they have a feeling of well-being and renewed vigour. As a result they stop worrying their physicians.

The effects of mental stress on total health will be seen more clearly when we discuss homoeostatis.

Chapter 6

Posture and Motion

Osteopathic interest in the posture of a patient is twofold.

First, an osteopath is concerned with the overall posture. This includes the *condition* of the muscles and their role as supporting structures with a function similar to the pillars which hold up a building. As the body has to be raised up these need power to overcome resistance and some may need to act as splints to hold the body erect. Posture also includes the characteristics of the skeleton and the condition of the joints, particularly longstanding or recent joint restrictions such as osteopathic lesions. A patient's way of life will without doubt have influenced their present posture as will have their occupation, their childhood physical development and inherited characteristics, as well as any accidents which may have befallen them. It is important for the osteopath to know to what extent postural influences brought about the condition of the muscles and joints as well as the complaint which led the patient to seek osteopathic advice.

Second, the osteopath is concerned with the effects which posture has had or is likely to have in the future upon the health of the patient.

Occupation
Occupation is one of the chief factors which affect the posture of modern man. Unnatural activities at work involve both mental and physical concentration. By physical concentration I mean sustained effort of the muscles which are working even when sitting or standing still. Low back muscles, for example, are

working when someone is typing or book-keeping and neck and head muscles are working when minding a machine, even though they are not the muscles directly involved in the activity. In fact most muscles of the body are involved in any task. Strain is placed upon the muscles from postural attitudes and the body always automatically tries to counteract these by continuous movement of the neck, trunk, legs or head etc. If this counteracting process did not occur the body would sag. Sometimes these counteracting processes are inadequate to reduce strain, so rapid changes in posture occur. The amount of work done by muscles when holding the body in a fixed position is greater than in many active physical pursuits.

Normal muscle work when performed regularly, and especially for pleasure, is good for the health of the body. When muscles work to perform any movements they do so by contracting rather like a telescope and muscle fibres shorten and widen. This contraction is effected by impulses which travel down nerve fibres and these fibres need food in the form of oxygen which is supplied by the blood. Extra contraction will, of course, need extra blood and sustained work will induce fatigue. Because extra blood is needed there is an increase in the production of waste products (carbon dioxide, lactic acid etc.) which must be disposed of in the blood-stream through the veins and lymph for excretion in the urine. Muscle contraction needed for concentrated physical attention will cause these waste products to accumulate too quickly in the muscle fibres and bring about muscle fatigue. When waste products stagnate within a muscle whose blood supply is not sufficient to provide oxygen and drain waste products away, stiffening of the muscles is soon experienced. If this is an habitual experience actual restriction of the joints will ensue. When the body is continuously held in one particular position for perhaps a period of years it will adapt to its environment and the stance of the individual will change to accommodate the situation, with the ultimate outcome of a greatly altered posture. Even the bones, as we have explained, will adapt over a period of years to the mould of their environment and postural changes become almost irreversible.

Inherited factors

We acquire inherited physical characteristics from both parents and the build which we inherit has a lot of bearing upon our posture. Although we may not develop the same postural habits as our parents, or have the same lifestyle, our basic bone structure will impose postural problems which they have had. 'Somatyping' is one system of classifying physique. This method is based upon the work of William Sheldon who recognized three types of body structure: the endomorph, the mesomorph and the ectomorph. This classification is essentially concerned with shape and not size. According to Sheldon each one of us has a modicum of all three in our basic structural frame. These structural types may very well have ethnological origins and in remoter parts of the world where there have been few territorial changes and little history of subjugation by invaders, varieties of structural type are less evident.

We will compare two types of structure which, for simplicity we will describe as 'thin' types and 'stocky' types (see Figure 4). *A 'thin' type does not mean someone undernourished but an individual with a thin elongated bone structure.* Such a person will have deeper curves in the spine as a result of having long, thin muscles and therefore weaker support. A tall 'thin' type often develops a stoop. The body leans backward and the chest is inclined to be flat and because of this the shoulders may droop. 'Thin' types, are usually more flexible than the stocky type. Modern life does not require any of us to use fully and regularly all our muscles and ligaments for everyday activities and so predisposes postural problems. Because of their physical characteristics, 'thin types' are more vulnerable to these influences.

Inside the structure of the 'thin' type the organs are found to be drawn downward, which is not the ideal 'normal'. Because the chest sags the diaphragm will be in a lower position as will the heart which rests upon it and the liver, stomach and spleen immediately beneath.

The 'stocky' types, on the other hand, with thicker bones and muscles, usually have shorter ligaments and are not so flexible. They do not, as a general rule, develop a tendency towards

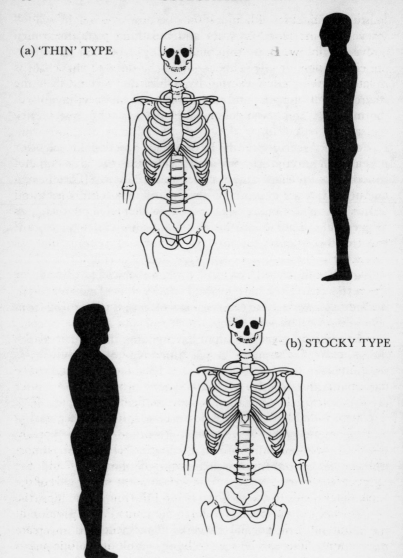

Figure 4. Classification of bone structure: (a) 'thin' type; (b) 'stocky' type.

postural difficulties although if they become overweight will fall prey to heart, blood-pressure and breathing problems which inevitably follow. Both 'thin' and 'stocky' types can, of course, be either short or tall. This is nothing to do with shape but is related to the control exerted by the pituitary gland over the thyroid and gonads and the release of a specific growth hormone. A 'thin' type does not become a 'stocky' type or vice versa.

For many years those who have studied functional reasons for disease have compiled evidence to show that the 'thin' type of person is considerably more susceptible to disease. They have a greater incidence of gastric disorder, influenza, bronchitis and colitis as well as being more prone to mental illness such as depression. They also have a greater tendency toward structural disorder for the very obvious reason that as 'structures' they are less compact and the external forces which bring about injury such as 'disc' problems are more difficult for them to resist. They have longer body levers and weights lifted, including the weight of their own trunk, are further away from the fulcrum upon which they pivot.

The 'stocky' type, naturally having less movement of the joints, much thicker muscles and stronger, shorter ligamentous attachments, are less vulnerable to the factors that induce osteopathic lesions. Ironically, however, when they do suffer such problems they are usually more difficult to relieve.

Those individuals who develop bad posture whether during their formative years or time spent at work are, if their posture worsens, most likely to suffer osteopathic lesions. An almost predictable susceptibility to disease will ensue. Should the posture so change as to throw the weight of the upper part of the spine backwards to the position behind the line of the hips, the strain would be so great as to force the joints into a position at the limit of their normal range of movement and so create restrictions. This can be seen to be the result of a subtle *process* which may have been continuing over a number of years (see Figure 5).

Postural changes bring about shortening and contraction of

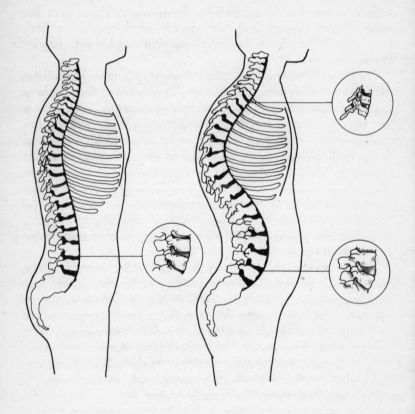

Figure 5.   Bad posture causing joint restriction and wedging of
               discs.

muscles which will reduce the normal range of the joints and so the range through which they are regularly taken in everyday use becomes their normal limit. If taken beyond that range the joints will be strained and an osteopathic lesion will be induced. Should the action be sudden, injury to the intervertebral disc may result:

Structural Anomalies

Dr Still once asked the question, 'does a bone construct its own habitation?' The answer is clearly a positive 'Yes'. This is confirmed when there has been some minor disorganization of the position of a joint, for instance the hip, during childhood. The development and shape of the joint itself is dependent upon mechanical factors, and muscular imbalance and disturbed symmetry of the structure will result from impeded function of the muscles.

A very large number of people have one leg shorter than the other. If this leg has grown shorter during their early development as a child then progressive deformity of the skeleton will have taken place. The spinal column will have formed in an environment of tension which has forced it to lean over to one side at the base and curve higher up in order to compensate (see Figure 6). A permanent lateral curvature (scoliosis) will result from this and the supporting muscles on each side of the spine will have unequal development. This condition never corrects itself and the deformity will often increase, especially if an unsuitable occupation is chosen. Muscular distortion and the contraction of ligaments is particularly common in tall thin subjects.

Those with such anomalies as a short leg are also much more likely to be candidates for osteopathic lesions and are particularly susceptible to trouble in the low back, mid back and neck, frequently suffering recurrences of severe problems in these areas.

These osteopathic lesions may similarly cause acute physical symptoms such as pain and restriction with all the other complementary factors. Sometimes the condition will become

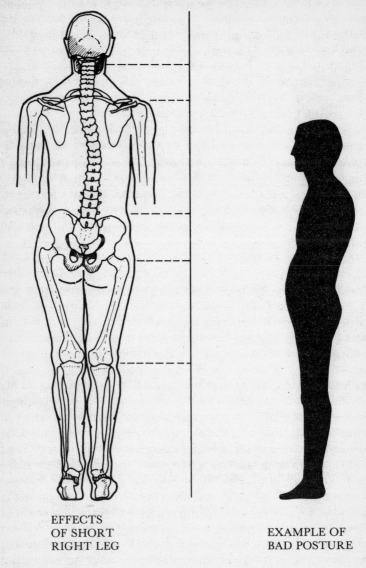

EFFECTS
OF SHORT
RIGHT LEG

EXAMPLE OF
BAD POSTURE

Figure 6.   The effects on the spine of a short right leg.

chronic if not rectified quickly and often the total body structure will adapt to accommodate it. A permanent irreversible postural and mechanical change will then persist. Inflammatory processes may develop in the joints, with referred pains in the abdominal area from irritated nerve roots. Because of the far reaching effects of osteopathic lesions other painful symptoms may arise in the vicinity of the gall bladder, the spleen, the lower abdomen and the appendix, for example.

There are other ways, of course, that a patient may have acquired a shortening of a leg. One very obvious cause could be the result of an accident in which a leg was badly broken and so shortened in repair. When this happens the body is forced to compensate by its own adjustment bringing imbalances and stress into the structure. A marked shortening of a leg will generally result in unnatural wear on the hip joint and so precede pathological conditions such as arthritis.

Should it be that some deformity of the foot occurred at birth or developed during childhood then all the problems mentioned will develop with growth and become permanent postural features to which the child will adapt. This is a problem that orthopaedic consultants and physiotherapists involved in pediatrics have for long been concerned with. They, too, regard the correction of faults in posture of children of considerable importance.

Bad posture, especially that which is brought about by prolonged occupational habits, can easily be seen to have adverse effects upon the organs of the body and result in ill health. The function of any organ of the body may be influenced: the liver, the kidneys, the lungs, the colon or even the heart. Postural changes which alter the carriage of the chest will interfere with the action of the diaphragm, thereby impeding breathing, and will have an adverse effect upon the thoracic and abdominal veins that pass through it, which in turn will produce congestion of blood in the pelvis and lower abdomen. A downward drag will ensue involving the stomach, the nerves which come from the heart and other nerves arising in the neck. Apart from physical strain on the heart, interference with its nerve supply higher up will doubly involve it. These postural problems when combined with the detrimental effects of osteopathic lesions, which they may even have brought about, can be identified as the initiating cause of an endless list of common disorders, one of the most frequently experienced being gastric disturbance.

Each individual has a postural 'normal' in which he/she functions quite adequately, even with mechancial defects, but some people whose posture is bad are more vulnerable than others. The incidence of osteopathic lesions which put strain upon the supporting structures and create restriction of motion are sufficient to tip the delicate balance between the individual's best easy normal and a condition of impeded mobility that is the first step towards ill health.

Bound up with these problems of posture are the conditions that arise when the actual anatomical relationships of internal organs are disturbed. As we have shown, very minor disorganization of any structure can begin a process that can lead to illness. When an organ such as the diaphragm, the liver, or the gall bladder is very marginally displaced distressing symptoms can appear. One very clear example of this situation will be seen by studying the duodenum. This structure lies next to the pancreas and part of it is subject to pressures from sections of the small intestine. As the duodenum is a tube it can easily be closed by external pressure. This tube may also kink if affected by downward drag on adjacent structures, with gastric disturbances the obvious outcome.

This very brief discussion of postural problems should illustrate Dr Still's principle that the body is a unit and that abnormal structure or function in one part exerts abnormal influence on other parts (see Figure 7). This is why osteopaths find it fundamental to recognize the type of individual they are examining and so form a conception of the shape and size of the skeleton, the type of joints, the position of the viscera and the mechanical behaviour of the patient. To consider any treatment without this approach would at best be palliative. The malady for which the patient seeks help is usually the tip of the iceberg

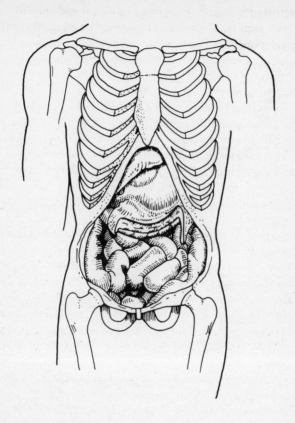

Consideration of the close
anatomical relationships of the
internal organs shows how
postural changes must cause them
to be compressed and displaced
from 'normal' positions

Figure 7. The close relationships of the internal organs mean that
postural changes cause the organs to be compressed and
displaced from 'normal' positions.

and treatment of, say, back pain without considering all the inducing factors would be poor osteopathy and unlikely to bring any lasting benefit.

Chapter 7

Fascia and Effect of Strain

Although the formation of the bone structure and the condition and health of the ligaments, tendons and muscles are most important factors that govern the amount of success with which postural balance is coped with, the importance of the fascia must not be overlooked.

In studying textbook anatomy there is a tendency to split the structures of the body into clearly defined parts in order to identify their separate functions. This is a very necessary exercise, but to grasp the osteopathic approach it is a prerequisite to understand that an interplay between *all* physical structures is necessary to produce the free *motion* which is essential to good health. Osteopathic training includes biomechanics and kinesiology as well as anatomy and physiology.

All the tissues which hold the body together and support it must be pliable and resilient. If for any reason they lose their pliability or resilience, as for instance they might if immobility or tension occurred, there will be many losses of efficiency in the functions they perform and not only can the movement of the major structure of the body be disabled but also the internal health-regulating processes.

As an example let us briefly examine the fascia of the pelvis. Many layers of fascia cover the surface of the pelvis and wrap around the veins and arteries. In the lower part of the abdomen they reinforce the action of the muscles and the ligaments. The fascia forms a network which sometimes supports the organs, muscles and bones and at other times protects them. It is a dense glittering sheath which in one place may be tight, in another loose and web-like, sometimes thicker where areas of extra strength and protection are needed. It lies in between muscles and forms a buffer which is so strong that it actually serves as the origin of many muscles and increases their power.

Pelvic Strains

There is one particular band of fascia in the pelvis known as the *fascia lata* that acts as a sheath to all the muscles of the thigh, covers the whole of the back of the pelvis and extends through to the muscles of the lower abdomen. It goes down as far as the knee, over which it passes and interweaves with the fascia of the lower leg. At the side of the thigh it forms the very strong attachment for the most important muscle the *tensor fascia lata* (see Figure 8). The function of this muscle is to tighten the entire sheath of the fascia lata and to rotate the thigh inwards slightly as well as lift it. The fascia is wrapped around the thigh muscles and prevents any individual muscles from overworking, so ensuring safe movement of the hip.

Any restriction of the hip joint, the knee joint, the pelvic joints or even the lower lumbar spine will immediately produce incapacitating symptoms over the entire extent of the fascia lata and every part it serves and supports. Within the pelvis, as we have seen when there is hip shift, the consequential strains on organs, arteries and veins will encourage insidious effects.

Cells

What we should now consider is a much more subtle and more serious possibility; namely, that loss of pliability and resilience in the tissues will impede their regenerative and reparative capacity. This is not just a matter of the chemistry of our bodies being able to synthesize products necessary for continuing health. It involves the very important matter of *movement*; not just movement of the bones, muscles, tendons, ligaments and fascia or the blood in the arteries and veins adjacent to them but

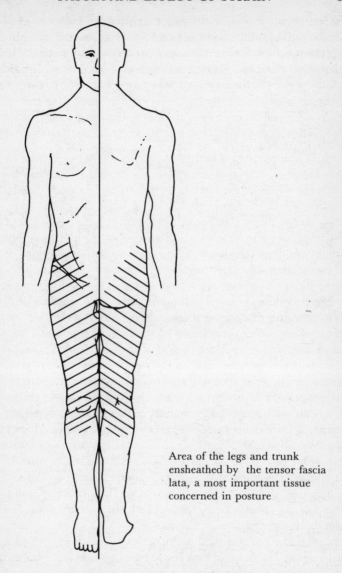

Area of the legs and trunk
ensheathed by the tensor fascia
lata, a most important tissue
concerned in posture

Figure 8.   Area of the legs and trunk ensheathed by the tensor
fascia lata.

the *movement of cells*. Cells must be free to move in order to
perform their duty as agents for the normal repair and
replacement of tissue elements necessary to cope with the
everyday wear and tear of our physical activities. Should the
fascia lose its open texture, which it could do if continually
strained, and become progressively less resilient, the movement
of the cells will be gradually impeded. Conditions of disease will
arise if the body is unable to adapt to compensate adequately for
this failure.

Dr Still recognized and emphasized the danger:

> I have thought for many years that the lymphatics and cellular
> system of the fascia.... do get filled with impure and unhealthy
> fluids, long before any disease makes its appearance and that the
> procedure of changes known as fermentation, with its electro
> magnetic disturbances, were the cause of a high percentage of the
> disease that we labour to relieve.

For a striking example of the importance of fascia in relation
to health and disease let us now look at the neck.

Neck Strains
Quite apart from the roots of the nerves (see Chapter 5) which
emanate from the spinal cord, there is another nervous system
known as the autonomic system, whose parts are commonly
described as the sympathetic and parasympathic systems. The
possibilities of disturbance of this system are endless. It not only
supplies all the secretory glands and many muscles known as
'smooth' but it is concerned with all the numerous bodily
functions which are involuntary in action, such as those of the
stomach and intestines, alterations of the calibre of the blood
vessels, the beat of the heart and the maintenance of the
metabolic processes.

The main portion of this system consists of a series of nerve
cell stations situated in two rows, one on each side and in front
of the spinal column. One of the most important parts of this
system (the cervical ganglion) is found within the neck and

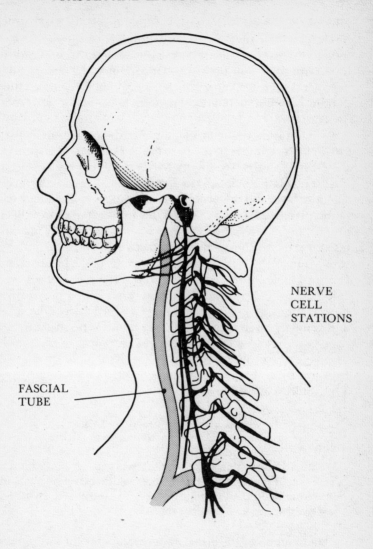

NERVE
CELL
STATIONS

FASCIAL
TUBE

Figure 9. Part of the sympathetic nervous system in the neck, showing the close relationship to the bones and fascial tube.

innervates the blood vessels of the head, as well as such important structures as the sweat glands of the head and the muscle fibres that dilate the eye. It has connections with important nerves in the neck. Disturbances in this part of the nervous system are known to cause emotional responses such as fainting, crying, palpitation and diarrhoea, and it also reacts to infections.

Lying in front of the spinal bones of the neck is an important fascia that originates in the base of the skull and is suspended in the form of a tube (see Figure 9). This tube of fascia is fixed to the front of the spine by a ligament just below the neck at shoulder level and then continues in another form to the bottom of the rib cage. Passing through this tube at the side of the neck are sheaths of arteries supplying blood to the head. This tube of fascia performs the vital and sensitive work of adapting and stabilizing all the complicated movements of the head and neck. If disturbances of the position of the vertebrae were allowed to continue, and a postural adaptation result, a host of disorders of the functions of the body would probably arise. The arteries and veins themselves are very close to the bone structure. Both poor posture and osteopathic lesions can cause tension in these vessels and so interfere with the circulation of the head. Pressure from the fascia can impede blood flow.

Dr Still's conclusion was,

> The part the fascia takes in life and death gives us one of the greatest problems to solve. It surrounds each muscle, vein, nerve and all organs of the body. It has a network of nerve cells and tubes running to and from it … it is crossed and no doubt filled with millions of nerve centres and fibres which carry on the work of secreting and excreting fluids, vital and destructive. By its action we live and by its failure we die.

The freedom of the circulation throughout the entire body is also only ensured if the fascia is in an easy condition of tone. A healthy tone aids the muscles, ligaments and tendons which in turn aid the balance of the body. The condition of one is dependent upon the other and so the bones, muscles, tendons, ligaments and fascia act as a harmonizing team.

Chapter 8

Homoeostatis

Every cell of the human body lives in fluid known as extra-cellular fluid. This bathes the minute spaces between the cells and is carried from one part of the body to another in the blood.

This extra-cellular fluid is made up of constituents which are provided through the function of almost every organ of the body. The lungs, for instance, bring oxygen from the air into the blood, which transports it to all the tissues and cells. The digestive system absorbs nutrients from the food in the blood. The endocrine glands and the liver convert nutrients for the digestive system into substances that can be used by the cells and so on. The blood-stream is, therefore, the place in which all these substances are mixed and maintained at the correct constancy to provide good health. It was an American physiologist Walter Cannon who described this maintenance of constant conditions of the fluid as 'homoeostatis'. For the body's cells to survive, the composition of their surrounding fluids must be precisely maintained at all times.

Dr Still described the organs of the body as 'functionaries' with individual responsibilities and said,

> The human body as a whole is a functionary with duties to perform. The brain is a functionary whose duty is to prepare and send forth *through* the agency of the nervous system the forces and fluids necessary to the action of organs of the whole system, none excepted, and that function must be performed to the degree of *healthy perfection*.

Physiologists agree that homoeostatis is disturbed by stress, which in this sense means any stimulus that creates an imbalance in the extra-cellular fluid. Stress may come from such factors as heat, cold, loud noises or lack of oxygen or may occur within the body itself from pain, tumours, destructive emotions etc. Most stresses are mild but extreme stresses might arise from such factors as severe infection, surgical operations, overexposure and so forth.

The body has a remarkable ability to bring the extra-cellular fluids back into balance by means of regulating devices described as homoeostatis. Very high resistance to stress is often seen, and humans can adapt to extremes of environment such as high altitudes, desert heat and artic cold, for example. The nervous system detects when the body is deviating from its balanced state and, by sending messages to the appropriate organs to counteract stress, works to regulate homoeostatis.

Dr Still explained, when discussing one important organ,

> Should this functionary fail to receive the proper force from the nervous system it is to be expected that the arterial blood will be of an impure and inferior quality. Thus all organs will show disease in proportion to the quality of arterial blood upon which they are fed and from which they receive nourishment.

Life within the human body is then rather like a stream which flows into a pool at one end and out at the other. So long as that flow (motion) is uninterrupted, the water in the pool will be clear and fresh. Outgoing water would make space for incoming water which would provide sustenance for the life which thrived in it and there would be homoeostatis. Should the outward flow be obstructed there would be no current through the pool and its water would become stagnant; incoming fresh water would encounter a slimy bog, from which the outflow would become dirty and trickling.

Consider the chief processes of life; we must breathe in fresh oxygen and breathe out carbon dioxide as well as other vaporized wastes. We need food to rebuild the cells of the body and provide energy; this is achieved with the help of oxygen. Waste products from the muscle tissues and cells are rejected into the blood and lymph and discharged from the body. The bowels and urinary system are the outlets for waste. Thus the human disgestive system works in a similar way to the pool we have discussed.

The pores of the skin, too, are essential for the absorption of the effects of light, air and water and themselves give off waste by means of perspiration.

It is, therefore, vitally important to keep all these outlets of elimination actively open. When there are injudicious living habits they inevitably become clogged and their actions sluggish with the result that the bowel, kidney, lungs and skin become stagnant in the same way as a stream. Eventually the blood cells, stomach, liver and intestines will in turn be congested by accumulating waste such as acids, toxins and irritant poisons, and these will be reabsorbed in the blood itself. In such a way the homoeostatic forces of the body will suffer stress and their function will be impaired. Symptoms of catarrh, colds, influenza, bronchitis, headaches, kidney and liver disorder, and possibly arthritis, will develop. These will only be occasional in the beginning and may manifest themselves as short acute crises. They will be signs that the body is attempting to reject the waste products. If the symptoms are temporarily suppressed by drugs and nothing done to alter the habits that produce them, however, they will become chronic conditions which may only be controlled by palliatives.

We have discussed in Chapter 7 how fascial strain can impede the important movement of cells and how gastric disorders arise from bad posture. It is clear also that structural restrictions such as osteopathic lesions will contribute to ill health by altering homoeostatic processes and, in particular, perhaps interfere with the nerve supply not only to the organs but to the mechanisms that regulate homoeostatis.

Another aspect of homoeostatic constancy being affected by stress is in the form of psychological repression, arising perhaps from fear and anxiety. This can be maintained by muscular tension in any part of the body. Much vital energy is repressed by muscular tightness. This brings needless fatigue and tiredness as muscle groups, which should be alternately tensed and relaxed, vie against each other. It may also lead to osteopathic lesions. Not until these lesions are released and muscular and mental tension relaxed can easy mobility be regained. Relaxed breathing, heartbeat and digestive functions can then be restored and enjoyed, and suppleness of the spine and limbs will follow. Thinning and hardening of the inter-vertebral discs will be less likely to develop if the downward drag of gravity is lessened by improved posture.

We may reasonably accept that a variety of factors can influence homoeostatis and that it has a great ability to make the adjustments needed to cope with disturbing processes. However, once imbalance has occurred it is not easy to restore equilibrium and if body fluids are not quickly brought back into balance ill health will arise. To correct only one contributory cause of disturbance is not enough. If a person, for example, with a gastric ulcer, back pain, headaches and poor posture induced by occupation were to become chronically ill there would be no success in simply treating the ulcer problem in an isolated way. The release of osteopathic lesions, a re-education programme of exercises, treatment with muscle and organ relaxation techniques, including some self-applied ones, would all be necessary in addition to the obvious rearrangement of diet essential to assist healing. And so we return to the idea of treating the whole person and all his/her problems rather than simply the presenting symptoms, along with the necessity to appreciate that disorder in one part of the body is not unrelated to disorder in another.

Chapter 9
Disc Injuries

One of the most perplexing problems for patients is to understand the multitude of diagnostic descriptions they are given for their 'disc' complaints and to reconcile one practitioner's description of their condition with that of another. Descriptions include bulging discs, worn discs, disc lesions, shrinking discs, cracked discs, strained discs, compressed discs, degenerated discs and, of course, the most commonly used, slipped discs. A very great number of patients believe that discs 'come out' and that osteopaths, by some special means known only to them, 'put them back "in" ' again. 'Slipped disc' is not an osteopathic term although it has entered osteopathic terminology, having been used so frequently by general medical practitioners and other practitioners of physical medicine as well as the media for many years. The term has the value of being a simple way of explaining to a patient that they have a disc problem without concerning them with too much detail and at the same time assuring them that they are not suffering from a much more serious complaint which the acute and distressing disc symptoms may cause them to fear. Unfortunately, 'slipped disc' has so often been interpreted literally to imply that a disc has 'slipped' as if it could be separated from the joints of the spine. The term 'slipped disc' has also become synonymous with 'prolapsed disc' in many quarters. This again has made it difficult for patients to understand diagnosis, followed by much misrepresentation of how osteopathic treatment is applied to the condition.

I will try to clarify the problems of diagnosis of disc injuries and back problems related to them as well as explain the osteopathic approach to their treatment.

Causes

There are basically two main causes for disc problems. The first is the almost predictable outcome of continuing imbalances in the posture of the body and, in particular, the effects of an imbalanced pelvis. These imbalances can be inherited or acquired by gradual development or accident. In other words, many disc injuries have the same basic causes as osteopathic lesions and are, therefore, identifiable with a *continuing process* of stress and strain which ultimately causes the spinal joints to give way when some very ordinary movement of the body tips the balance of the forces that support the spine. Any of the factors mentioned in Chapters 4 and 6 on osteopathic lesions or posture may contribute to or induce a disc injury. In many of these cases osteopathic lesions are present before a disc injury occurs and patients may have suffered some back pain and restriction for some time beforehand. *This is another most important reason why osteopathic lesions should be found and released at an early date.*

The second main cause of disc injury is severe and sudden strain.

Structure of Discs

The structure of an intervertebral disc is popularly shown to be a pad which acts as a shock absorber between the bodies of the vertebrae. This is true but it should be emphasized that the disc is made out of thick fibro-cartilage, surrounded by a laminated portion and that it *grows* out of one bone and into another. It is not separate and each disc is firmly attached to a long powerful ligament which extends the full length of the front of the spine from the pelvis to the head and is similarly attached to another such ligament at the back of the spine. These, together with the bones, discs, tendons and fascia, make the whole spine a working unit. The idea, then, that pads slip out is very misleading and must not be taken literally. In fact, during adolescence the bones of the spine are much more likely to give way when subjected to violence than the discs, provided there are none of the signs of weakening which I shall mention later.

If you could cut through a disc you would see that its construction is rather like a squashed golf ball. The outside consists of laminated fibrous tissue known as the *anulus* fibrosus, and the inside of a softer tissue known as the *nucleus* pulposus. It is essential to realize that there is a considerable change in the pliability of the disc as a person ages. This is because the inside or nucleus changes with age. At birth the pliable tissues occupy a large area. As age advances these tissues are gradually replaced by stronger fibro-cartilage and the difference between the outside and the inside structures is much more difficult to distinguish, so much so that in old age it would require a microscope to detect the difference in structure of the nucleus.

Some time after the age of thirty and usually well before the age of forty, a gradual process of desiccation of the disc begins and there is a progressive loss of elasticity in the disc from then onwards. Discs will, therefore, usually be narrower in old age as a consequence of the loss of fluid in the joints which progressively decreases.

It is not uncommon, however, for a narrowing of a single disc to occur at a relatively early age. These younger cases are most probably due to the early occurrence of an osteopathic lesion induced by problems of abnormal postural balance. Occasionally they may have been caused by childhood injury.

Unnatural narrowing or shrinkage of a disc can arise from the presence of an osteopathic lesion at any time during its normal pliable life. When a slight yielding of the joint occurs within a normal range of movement and a fixing of the articulation of the bone exists for a long time, the joint will be deprived of nutrition and the tissue fluids will be restricted. The elasticity of the discs is known to depend upon the fluid content and, if osteopathic lesions persist, the joints will inevitably become more vulnerable to stresses and strains. In certain circumstances they will give way, causing further injury to the joint itself.

Some Types of Disc Injury

To help patients understand the diagnosis of disc problems we
will look at some of the different kinds of disc injury.

Locking of Facets

The very commonest of all back disorders involving discs is
caused through *jamming or locking of the facets of the spinal bones*.
When this happens the difference between the degrees of
restriction and the severity of the symptoms are very wide. If
you study Figure 10 you will see that the articular process of the
top bone, which should fit into and articulate with the grooves
of the articular process of the lower bone, has shifted. The
adjacent muscles, ligaments, tendons and fascia are all involved
in a tensioning reaction and so are holding the bones in an
abnormally fixed position. The muscles will have instinctively

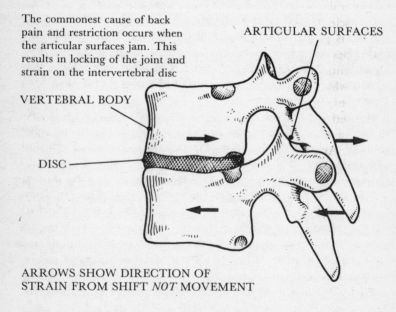

The commonest cause of back
pain and restriction occurs when
the articular surfaces jam. This
results in locking of the joint and
strain on the intervertebral disc

ARTICULAR SURFACES

VERTEBRAL BODY

DISC

ARROWS SHOW DIRECTION OF
STRAIN FROM SHIFT *NOT* MOVEMENT

Figure 10. The commonest cause of back pain and restriction
occurs when the articular surfaces jam.

contracted to protect the joint from further injury and will be guarding it, thereby increasing limitation of general movement. The disc itself is not displaced but will be strained at the attachment to the bones above and below and also strained at the attachment to the long ligaments that support the spine and which are attached to each vertebra. The amount of contraction will depend entirely upon the amount of shift that has occurred.

This condition is almost identical to an osteopathic lesion. It is almost, but not quite, the same and can produce similar, but not exactly the same, symptoms to varying degrees. The difference is mainly that the disc has been hurt as a result of the incident that caused the condition. The symptoms will not be as subtle because, when the strain happened, the attached ligaments, tendons, muscles and fascia would have been *suddenly* hurt in a more *traumatic* way. All these adjacent tissues will generally be inflamed and other symptoms such as swelling and muscle tearing may occur.

What is perhaps most important to understand is that very rarely does one single joint give way under stress without some co-incidental strain on other parts of the body in the immediate area to which the joint is directly or indirectly connected. In some cases, parts of the body some distance from the injury can be affected. This is logical when one considers that ligaments and fascia attached to the pelvis are also attached to the base of the skull. Anyone with a back injury will have experienced the pains and pulling sensation felt in the lower back when they move their head forward for example.

All the symptoms which accompany an osteopathic lesion may arise, such as pain, numbness, pins and needles, sciatica etc. The pelvis more often than not is affected when lower lumbar bones are restricted, as is also the hip joint. Either of these may, in fact, have been previously restricted parts that brought about the lumbar strain.

Once you apply the postural implications mentioned in Chapter 6 you will see that the symptoms in almost every case are varied. A short 'stocky' person may suffer more muscle spasm than a tall 'thin' person; similarly a physcial worker with strong muscles may experience more pain from contraction and muscle guarding than an office worker. With only a very minor movement of a joint a person who has a very inflexible structure with short ligaments may experience more sciatic pain than a flexible outdoor type.

Patients will appreciate then that it is not a simple matter to decide how much injury has occurred within the joint or, if dealing with a less serious disc problem, how much movement has taken place. One patient may have acute symptoms and not suffered much injury, while another may have greater damage within the disc itself and not such acute symptoms.

Strained Discs

Another minor disc injury takes place when there has been an accident which caused the joint to move but then immediately return to its normal position. Then a *strain on the disc* occurs without any displacement. This could produce symptoms of strain or minor tearing in the attached ligaments as well as a short spell of nerve pain. All these symptoms could diminish almost entirely without treatment within a period of seven days and the strain heal.

Narrowing of Disc Space

I have explained how the discs begin a process of degeneration as an individual gets older and how other degeneration is brought about. X-rays often reveal a *narrowing* or *thinning* of the space between the joints when compared with earlier records. When this is discovered patients are usually told that wear and tear has occurrred, which may be depressing, especially if they are around or below middle age. The degeneration may have developed from a series of minor restrictions causing loss of nutrition in the joint. Frequently correct osteopathic treatment can bring about relief of symptoms. If there is a weakening of the joint it can be expected that further problems may recur from time to time. That X-ray evidence suggests degeneration in one disc is not necessarily too serious; some of it may be natural and, unless it is very advanced, it need not always be the chief cause of the symptoms which may be due more to locking of the facets of the joints.

All the descriptions such as shrinking discs, worn discs and narrowing discs relate to and arise from disc degeneration. An X-ray film which shows the space between two vertebrae to be narrower than adjacent joints may not be evidence of degeneration if there is no previous X-ray record with which to compare it, particularly if the general structure of the joint surfaces appears to be healthy. A simple case of uneven spacing or postural abnormality might exist and although it may have contributed to an injury need not be the prime cause.

Strained Ligaments
Ligaments and *tendons* can also be strained or sprained when joints have shifted. These also will heal with rest and any osteopathic treatment would be designed to assist healing. After the ligaments or tendons have healed, however, if pains or stiffness persist for sometime then it is likely that a restriction of the joint has occurred and needs to be released before the patient can become completely better. Healing of any minor injury to the disc will follow.

Binding of Joints
Another condition which is quite common, especially in those with sedentary occupations or inactive lives, is a *binding* of the joints due to lack of regular use. This binding can occur without any cause other than prolonged inactivity in the same way as machinery will seize up when not in use. Binding can cause many symptoms and when it occurs in more than one joint it is responsible for a considerable part of the aches and pains suffered by modern man and may produce many of the effects of osteopathic lesions. If this condition is not of long duration it will respond well to osteopathic treatment and will also be greatly assisted by thoughtfully devised and controlled exercise over a long period. Binding will affect the supply of fluids to the local area and the nourishment needed by the discs.

When binding of the joints occurs suddenly it is usually due to the patient suffering some force from below the body through the legs and pelvis such as might occur, say, by jumping awkwardly off a low wall. In these cases there is more accurately a *compression* of the disc between the joints than a simple binding. This condition needs careful diagnosis and responds well to special osteopathic techniques. In these cases the pelvis itself will be affected and the force from below will generally cause a sacro-iliac problem which in turn will strain the lower part of the spine. The symptoms arising can be very severe and attempts to release the spinal joints will be unsuccessful without proper treatment of the pelvis and possibly the hip.

More Serious Injuries
The more serious injuries to discs can involve what could generally be described as a *protrusion*.

The incidence of protrusion of discs is, in fact, not as frequent as we are encouraged to believe. Much publicity has been given to this subject during the last twenty years with insufficient emphasis upon the many other conditions mentioned which are much more common. Illustrations of this problem in both periodicals and neo medical literature are somewhat misleading because they imply that large portions of the disc are pushed out from between the joints when in reality a very minute amount of the contents generally move.

A protrusion of a disc may occur when after many recurrences of joint injury a final and more stressful movement occurs, causing a part of the already degenerated disc to shift and impinge upon the spinal cord (see Figure 11). Alternatively a protrusion may occur during a powerful physical action; the joint gives way and the disc itself is *ruptured* and may bulge causing pressure upon the adjacent structures. This most commonly affects indirectly the roots of the spinal nerves. In this event the sufferer may never have had any back trouble before and may be physically strong.

A rupture of a disc is the commonest of the severe injuries and medically this is described as a *herniated* disc.

Much more rarely the internal contents of the disc, the softer

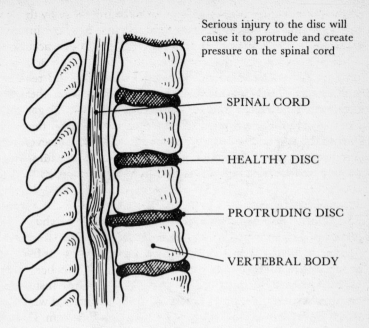

Serious injury to the disc will cause it to protrude and create pressure on the spinal cord

SPINAL CORD

HEALTHY DISC

PROTRUDING DISC

VERTEBRAL BODY

Figure 11. Serious injury to a disc will cause it to protrude and create pressure on the spinal cord.

tissue known as the nucleus, will extrude through a crack in the outside harder fibrous tissue, the annulus, and a prolapsed disc occur (see Figure 12). This may protrude into the spinal canal if the damage is at the back of the vertebra. You will gather from what has been said about the structure of a disc and the effects of the ageing process that a prolapsed disc will most likely be suffered by a person below middle age and more probably around thirty. That prolapses may occur earlier or later is relative to the physical health and medical history of the individual. After middle age the kind of injury that would induce a prolapse of a disc is likely to cause a protrusion of a hardened, or perhaps cracked, portion of a degenerated disc.

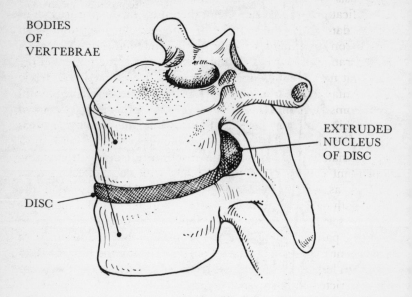

Figure 12. Example of serious prolapse.

Problems of Diagnosis of Disc Lesions

The family doctor when consulted by a patient suffering from disc symptoms is concerned with making a diagnosis which will assess the severity of the injury and enable him/her to make a decision as to what immediate action should be taken. The diagnostic methods used are perfectly satisfactory in so far as they indicate whether a severe injury exists, which requires immediate hospital supervision, or a less serious injury that may benefit from rest with further assessment later. Sometimes, as I have explained, there is a severe strain of the muscles or ligaments. When this has occurred it is unnecessary for any physical treatment to be administered and rest is the most common and sensible precaution. This initial method of diagnosis is not specific and does not necessitate the identification of the exact site of the injury or the precise extent of the damage to the joint before the general practitioner can advise on treatment to cope with immediate symptoms. A broad range of degrees of injury exists and some patients may feel that no advantage has been gained from forced rest, while others may feel that insufficient has been done to relieve painful symptoms. On the whole, however, the prevailing system of prescribing a short period of rest while the healing process begins is the best procedure in the early stages and most appropriately if a more serious disc injury exists. Osteopathic treatment can be given immediately with good effect in both serious as well as less serious injuries. However, what the osteopath decides to do will depend upon very careful diagnosis and in serious cases he may only give treatment designed to ease the patient's symptoms if he considers that another form of treatment may serve no useful purpose during the first ten days or so. In less severe cases he is likely to give treatment to release the restricted joints as soon as possible.

During the 1960s and 1970s it became common practice for many medical practitioners to write PID (prolapsed intervertebral disc) on medical certificates in nearly all cases where disc symptoms existed and, although these cases were not confirmed by orthopaedic consultants, a great many patients believed that they had suffered from prolapsed discs.

A large number of these patients obtained quick relief from osteopathic treatment and so a confusing situation developed which misrepresented the osteopathic profession as being able to cure such cases almost instantly. This brought disdain from the orthopaedic medical profession, who knew that such results were not possible, as well as confusion to many patients who became disillusioned with the results of previous medical treatment. The diagnosis of PID is now less widely used by GPs and has been replaced by the more appropriate description of 'disc lesion' which is preferable for all concerned and covers a wider variation in the degree of injury. The less serious disc injuries, then, do not involve any protrusion of the disc. All serious displacements are likely to do so, but only a small percentage result in prolapse.

The training that osteopaths receive to ensure competence in diagnosis of osteopathic lesions automatically provides them with a system of diagnostic techniques that are unrivalled in the assessment of disc injury and are unique in that they embrace the total physical condition of the patient. Even X-ray films, which are essential to eliminate suspected injury, or developing pathology provide little or no information about the disc injury that cannot be gained from a thorough osteopathic examination. No evidence as to whether there is actual movement between the joints can be found from an X-ray. It is not infrequent when minor deformities exist for an X-ray to lead a therapist to the wrong conclusion as to the site of the injury. Myelograms, too, have their limitations. They are essential to the surgeon to assess the exact position of a prolapsed disc but give no clue as to the amount of muscle tearing or contraction that has taken place or those factors which exist some distance from the site of the injury which may have a bearing upon its cause and possible recovery.

The osteopathic technique of testing for tension in the tissues is a valuable skill which can help diagnosis of severe disc conditions and often save a patient much discomfort by permitting early treatment.

Regular back sufferers know well the experience of sudden jabbing pains, which strike when only simple and minor movements have been performed such as lifting a cup or picking up a magazine. They know also how pain will develop either immediately, several hours later or possibly several days later. These are all very relevant details which the osteopath will need to know to enable him to make an accurate diagnosis. In nearly all cases there will have been a build-up of stress on the joint for some time due to postural imbalances or untreated osteopathic lesions. Even in cases of very sudden and severe injury to the disc the structure will have given way in the direction of the forces governed by the patient's posture and mechanical shape. The type and duration of the pain, the areas over which the pain travels, the amount of contraction in the muscles, and even such matters as the temperature of the surface of the skin will be important clues to accurate diagnosis. The patient's history of disc problems may reveal that the joint affected was the site of several previous incidents of strain and so predisposed to shift under stress. When a patient is suffering badly from pain and restriction the osteopath will not prolong their misery by carrying out a full osteopathic examination. However, at the first consultation he will need to satisfy himself about the extent of the injury and is not likely to start any treatment until he has done so.

Treatment of Disc Injuries

With very few exceptions all disc injuries of whatever kind or severity respond well to osteopathic treatment, and the less severe ones are quickly and effectively relieved. The more severe ones take longer depending upon the extent of the injury.

A very bad prolapse arising from a violent or traumatic accident will respond in the long term to osteopathic treatment but there are a few instances when osteopathic treatment will not relieve debilitating symptoms. In these cases surgery to remove part of the arch of the vertebra and the prolapsed disc is unavoidable.

The osteopathic belief is that surgery should not be contemplated until osteopathic methods have first been tried, unless the patient is suffering so much as to make the symptoms intolerable. A genuine prolapse cannot be *replaced* by any treatment of any sort for the obvious reason that the nucleus has extruded through a narrow split. However, specialized methods can relieve the pressure on the joint and assist healing. It has long been demonstrated that there are many cases of healed prolapse. The surrounding tissues have been shown to build up and form a new fibrous sheath around the extruded material. The process is believed to take between nine and twelve months, during which time the patient's mode of life will be restrained by the symptoms. This is, of course, a further reason for electing to undergo surgery.

Osteopathic treatment given during this period demands competent diagnosis of the level of injury and judicious application. Qualified osteopaths use special techniques for the treatment of prolapsed discs and they consider that any other type of manipulative treatment whatever is inadvisable once a prolapse has been confirmed.

Irrespective of the type of disc problem they have patients should never assume that their injuries are the same as their colleagues or fellow back sufferers simply because their symptoms appear to be the same. Careful osteopathic diagnosis will generally be able to forecast the expected results of proposed treatment and the time it will take.

When a patient has suffered a bad disc injury which has healed, fibrous adhesions will form around affected joints, these can initiate uncomfortable symptoms and need to be dispersed by osteopathic methods.

Apart from violent accidents no disc injury ever occurs without some predisposing physical causes. Those causes can be traced to the basic structure of the individual, his posture, occupation, social habits and physical history. It is osteopathic practice to attempt to identify those causes and, whenever possible, correct them by a programme of treatment combined with exercises and, where feasible, advice to alter the environmental conditions. In this way osteopathic management will contribute towards a more complete recovery as well as play a preventative role.

Chapter 10

Treatment

Before any treatment is contemplated an accurate diagnosis has to be made. In osteopathic terms this may not necessarily involve the naming of the condition, which is medically regarded as the label of the symptoms. An osteopath, being primarily concerned with mechanical faults, abnormalities of structure and restrictions of motion, will identify the causes of these irrespective of the resulting symptoms. Even so, a full and proper consultation must take place which requires the patient to give their medical history, details of all medication they are or have recently taken and their consulting physician's diagnosis of any complaint, whether they believe it relates to their osteopathic problem or not. An osteopath must decide whether any treatment is contra-indicated or needs modification. This is the one overriding reason why an osteopath must be adequately trained and the one justifiable reason why a physician should be cautious about referring a patient for manipulation to a particular practitioner.

Many patients have made up their own minds that they have 'disc' problems and may find that an osteopath may not readily accept their assessment without a full consultation. This is because backache may arise from such things as trouble in the stomach, gall bladder, kidneys or lungs, apart from muscular conditions, osteomyelitis, osteo-chrondritis, Paget's disease or a number of other diseases of the joint. Even when an osteopath is satisfied that such conditions do not exist the mechanical problems of the patient will be of importance when planning treatment and must therefore be identified. A good osteopath should recognize from experience when manipulation is unsuitable and because of his specialized training may very well see physical or joint problems that do not interest the family doctor because they would not be relevant to the type of treatment he would prescribe.

X-rays are not often necessary for osteopathic purposes and more significant information can be discovered by a physical examination. However, whenever an osteopath suspects the slightest possibility of any disease of the spinal column or other joints which would make his treatment unsuitable he will call for an X-ray before considering treatment. There are very rare circumstances when even X-rays may not show some condition that may make manipulation unsuitable but usually the patient will have had a history of symptoms which will have led to medical investigation much earlier or which the osteopath will have noted during his consultation. If by some extraordinary chance a patient has not consulted a family doctor about some symptoms that the osteopath feels need other specialized examination he will not give any treatment until he is satisfied about such problems. A patient may, therefore, consult a qualified osteopath with complete confidence.

An experienced and knowledgeable osteopath will use a wide range and variety of techniques in his daily work. He will vary his techniques as each situation demands and will also vary the length of treatment according to the patient's needs. An average treatment will take about twenty minutes to half an hour.

During the initial consultation the osteopath will have made an assessment of the basic needs of each patient as well as the presenting symptoms; an elderly patient, for example, would not be expected to dress quickly or be rushed during treatment; a patient with high blood-pressure or vertigo would not be asked to lie with their head held backward for any length of time; a patient with a very severe spasm of the deep muscles in the back would not be either examined or treated in a way which caused them undue aggravation of pain. Patients who are nervous or tense must be relaxed before any corrective treatment is contemplated. Even relaxed types of patients are often apprehensive of new experiences and so an osteopath will need to establish rapport with them.

Osteopathic treatment can never be standardized because individual treatment has to be created for each patient at a particular time to meet very individual conditions. The first thing a patient will notice when they visit a competent osteopath is that they have no equipment other than their own bare hands. If they have any electrical equipment it is because they are involved in some physiotherapy and probably specialize in treating superficial injuries, but they will not need it for osteopathic cases because it is completely unnecessary. Some osteopaths are also qualified as acupuncturists and may have pulse meters and such in their consulting rooms. They may sometimes use these in verifying a certain diagnosis. Treatment combining acupuncture has been found to be expedient in certain circumstances but both therapies are complete in themselves and should not be used together unless the practitioner has been fully trained in both. Dabbling in either acupuncture or osteopathic techniques is not beneficial and, indeed, may be harmful.

Osteopaths use what they call soft tissue treatments. These appear to the patient to be a kind of massage. Soft tissue treatment has no resemblance whatsoever, however, to the kind of massage provided in Turkish baths, gymnasiums or massage parlours. Neither is it similar to therapeutic massage used by trained masseurs; this has a different function. The kind of soft tissue treatment used by osteopaths is indeed exclusive to osteopathic training and is not used even by other types of manipulative therapists. The reason that osteopathy has developed soft tissue treatment is in consequence of Dr Still's teaching to 'look for and *begin* the treatment of all diseases in the fascia' which can only be influenced through the soft tissues. The techniques for soft tissue demand a certain flair which is not learned in a mechanical way, so the quality of soft tissue treatment varies from practitioner to practitioner. Soft tissue treatment when properly used can completely relieve many symptoms and so render such treatment as manipulation unnecessary.

The osteopath may consider it necessary to use a number of techniques for relaxing the patient, which involve gentle pressure on specific parts of the body, particularly the back, possibly involving breathing techniques. We think of a patient as being structurally 'in a tangle' and it is the job of the osteopath to disentangle the supporting structures. This could involve placing a patient in a number of different positions and using methods to synchronize breathing with gentle adjustment. The diaphragm or the neck could well receive attention. There are an endless variety of osteopathic treatments for reducing tension and preparing the patient for treatment with relaxed confidence. All the techniques mentioned should be found to be pleasant and comforting.

All the information which the osteopath has obtained during the initial consultation will be pertinent to the main treatment, which will be modified to suit the particular circumstances.

Attention will be given to all osteopathic lesions which have been detected. The joints affected will be located and very specific treatment used. The order of this treatment will be carefully worked out and no random movements of joints would ever be contemplated by a good osteopath. He is likely to release the joints which have most recently become restricted before any others and will have ensured that the proper preparation of the muscles and ligaments etc. has been made beforehand. It would be quite futile for any treatment of the sacro-iliac joint, for example, to be administered before problems of the lower back had been carefully assessed.

Whenever possible the osteopath will use gentle methods in preference to any manipulative techniques that involve the use of controlled force. These methods are sometimes described as 'functional' or as 'positional corrections'. A good osteopath would, under no circumstances, attempt to introduce movement into joints that have been restricted for a long time and it would depend upon the patient's requirements as to what he would advise as the best method of dealing with them. He might recommend a programme of corrective treatments using subtle stretching methods possibly combined with an exercise routine.

When lesions and altered postural balance have existed for some years they are regarded by osteopaths as chronic conditions which need careful management. No competent osteopath would attempt to correct such conditions quickly. To contemplate this would be foolish and harmful because attempted correction of one problem would inevitably lead to the development of further chronic conditions. This is why a good osteopath will explain long-standing causes and encourage the patient to consider postural management as well as a corrective exercise programme. Sudden movement of joints will not necessarily produce *natural motion* which is the ideal goal of osteopathic treatment.

A patient may find that the osteopath may minimize the amount of soft tissue work at the first treatment when dealing with acute conditions, even though it might be necessary to reduce spasm and possibly swelling near joints at a later stage. Patients often feel that they would like to have a 'good massage' but this may be inadvisable. Acute conditions are accompanied by inflammation which will reduce if the chief causative factors are relieved and so the osteopath is likely to attempt to release restricted joints first. Random manipulation in these cases is, however, quite definitely not suitable and might injure the soft tissues themselves. Osteopaths receive extensive training to ensure that the patterns which produced the lesions are properly diagnosed and that the most efficient method of relief is followed without aggravating symptoms to achieve successful results or occasioning the patient undue discomfort. In this they have a great advantage over non-osteopathic practitioners. Release from acute symptoms alone may seem to be a merciful relief to a distraught patient, but they should not ignore the need for further management if they wish to prevent the recurrence of the symptoms. It is sometimes better to suffer acute symptoms for a few days longer in order to achieve long-standing relief.

When employing manipulative techniques, the osteopath will

select 1 or 2 manoeuvres from as many as 150 alternatives. Here again he should adapt his treatment to the patient's needs. The shape and size of the patient will influence what he does. He will find it easier to use one technique on a very big patient and a completely different one on someone light, one technique on someone with a lateral curvature of the spine (scoliosis) and another on someone with a forward or backward curvature (kyphosis or lordosis), while older patients may need very different treatment. Many patients do not have very flexible structures and the osteopath will guard against taking, say a hip, beyond a comfortable range of movement. Osteopathic techniques are often easy to copy but are not effectively and safely carried out without training and experience.

Osteopathic manipulation has no connection whatsoever with surgical manipulation which is used for treating dislocations in hospitals. Any potential patient who has had a dislocation repositioned must not expect that osteopathic treatment is in any way similar.

The techniques used for moving joints and releasing osteopathic lesions are called by osteopaths 'adjustments'. This is the word which the profession finds most apt and is in fact an expression used extensively by Dr Still in his writings.

Although there are textbooks on osteopathic manipulative techniques and very specifically defined methods to use for each particular type of restriction, it is not or ever was the ideal of the osteopath to use a certain manipulation for the same restriction in different patients. The art of manipulation is rather like playing the piano; each player may be able to read the music but will inevitably give a different rendering of the tune. Musical critics can easily detect different presentations of the same concerto when played by virtuoso pianists. Patients undoubtedly do the same and will readily recognize a poor osteopath after having visited a good one. Furthermore, the best osteopaths will not be bound by specific treatments even when varied and modified to meet special needs but will devise their own methods of releasing joints. Thorough osteopathic training will have demanded a comprehensive knowledge of anatomy and will provide the basis for successful improvisation to achieve results.

Patients like to know if the treatment will hurt. Certainly manipulation should not do so. However, a certain amount of discomfort may be experienced for a moment when an adjustment is being made and this could be linked with a painful stimulus for a second or so. This will entirely depend upon the amount of pain the patient is suffering initially. No pain should ever be caused to a patient by osteopathic treatment when they do not present with a painful condition. If they are suffering acute pain on consultation it is quite unlikely that an osteopath will administer any treatment that will aggravate it. However, if a patient is in very acute pain he might find some of the techniques momentarily painful or uncomfortable. Because the osteopath may need to use the patient's body as a lever to release a restricted joint or move the patient through unusual positions to take the strain off joints concerned, the patient may feel as though they have been 'pulled about'. This feeling is also commensurate with the amount of discomfort or pain that they have in the first place and someone receiving treatment for a non-acute condition should find the entire treatment pleasant. The purpose of placing a patient in curled-up or slightly contorted position is, in fact, designed to take the joint through a range that will enable the osteopath to release it with the minimum amount of effort. Often joints can be released by placing the patient in an unusual position without any manipulation at all. Sometimes the osteopath will decide against the use of manipulation of joints altogether and employ other techniques such as stretching, rhythmic breathing or reflex treatment.

It has recently become habitual to describe osteopathic manipulation as a technique using a high velocity thrust. This is not an ideal generalization at all. The word thrust implies forcibly driving or pushing and is associated with forward-directed forces. There are a small number of manipulations where a very controlled sudden push is used, but this push is made through a very modified range and with specific intention. The patient feels a very short and sudden movement of specific joints. This may cause discomfort or slight pain for a split second only. It is much more likely to cause surprise if done expertly because the patient should be completely relaxed at the moment it is done. The majority of manipulations do not, however, involve this push-type technique and are more like passive movements used to release joints involving some leverage and some separating-type movements. A trained osteopath will not use 'sudden' methods unless the patient is both suitably and adequately prepared.

The amount of treatment that is given will depend first of all upon what the patient has asked the osteopath to deal with and, subsequently, upon what is considered necessary to get the patient better and then any management that seems advisable. If a patient declines management there will be no pressure from a busy practitioner. Osteopathic management is an entirely optional matter.

Should the patient have a longstanding illness the initial consultation may take up to one hour and some treatment might be given. The osteopath may suggest a programme of short treatments over a long period at widening intervals. From his experience he should be able to forecast the amount of treatment needed, but may not be able to do so precisely. In these cases the patient may reasonably expect the practitioner to give an approximation of what is needed and the costs involved. The patient may then decide whether they wish to undergo the treatment.

Where poor posture has been one of the chief causes of the complaint and sagging of the internal organs and structures of the body has become an aggravating factor, treatment will be very comprehensive. The treatment may involve techniques to relieve any mechanical blockage of the circulation, adjacent adhesions will be released, and methods to relieve congestion of the organs employed. The structures will be lifted by manual treatment and the osteopath will achieve this by using the pads of his fingers to manipulate through the soft tissues. The patient will probably be treated lying down, on the back, on the stomach or perhaps on the side.

When there is disturbed anatomical relationship specific techniques will be used. Some examples are drainage of the gall bladder, lifting of the colon, relaxing of the diaphragm, and relieving congestion in portal veins. During examination for these conditions the osteopath will have carefully tested the rhythms of the breathing mechanisms and noted any disharmony in primary patterns. Because these rhythms are bound up with the problem of balance and gravity the patient may be placed in unusual positions so that the osteopath may compare changes in the rhythmic effects.

As osteopathy is concerned with all causative factors the treatment will include the diagnosis and adjustment of any osteopathic lesions. It may include some manipulation of the spine and will certainly include general treatment of all structures that in any way, however remotely, affect the stresses on the organs concerned.

Chapter 11

Cranial Osteopathy

Cranial osteopathy is an advance in osteopathic medicine which has developed from the work of W.G. Sutherland, a student of Dr Still, and whose research began about fifty years ago. Dr Still himself stressed the importance of the total concept of osteopathic therapy and used many techniques which involved the treatment of the head of a patient as part of the treatment of the whole body. He also stated that the cerebro-spinal fluid was 'the highest known element in the human body' and sought to influence its action in healing.

Dr Sutherland, however, by first concentrating his attention upon the idea that the joints of the skull were intended for motion, made very crucial discoveries about the involuntary movements related to respiration that take place throughout the body, as well as the motion of the central nervous system and its connecting structures. The outcome of this was the development of a completely new range of diagnostic and treatment techniques which expanded the potential of osteopathic treatment. Although these related to treatment of the skull they broadened the total approach to mechanical causes of illness by reason of the relationships of the cranial mechanisms to the function of the rest of the body and homeostatis. These advances, in fact, highlighted the osteopathic belief that treatment should include the whole body as opposed to dealing with locally affected parts. Dr Sutherland's theory concerning the motion of the cerebro-spinal fluid has since been substantiated by modern scientific evidence.

The work that Dr Sutherland innovated has now crystallized into a section of osteopathic therapy which has enormous scope. Very few practitioners outside the USA have training in this type of treatment but there is a gradual expansion of interest in it by existing practitioners and more of its principles are being incorporated into early training. The techniques used require a high degree of palpatory skill and sensitive application. The very nature of the work precludes any forceful-type manipulative treatment and, as many infants can benefit from it, clearly all treatment must be extremely gentle and controlled. Cranial osteopathy is concerned with a physiological balance which osteopaths describe as the cranial mechanism. This mechanism may be out of rhythm or its equilibrium disturbed either from accident or an experience at birth which may have induced structural imbalances.

This book is not the place to go deeply into the theory of cranial osteopathy, however, and we will have to confine our interest to the disorders which have been shown to benefit from it. All these examples have been clinically tested with good results by cranial practitioners.

In both adults and children cranial treatment is most successful in dealing with symptoms resulting from direct trauma to the head. Often the incidents that caused the problems may have been forgotten by the patient because they recovered from them quickly and no hospital treatment was necessary. Consequently the presenting maladies are unconnected with the cause. Local pains, headaches, dizziness and nausea are symptoms that could reasonably be seen as likely to respond to cranial treatment. Others less obvious, such as fatigue, loss of appetite, possible anorexia and disturbances of vision may often benefit. Some of the most successful results have been obtained when treating small children. Problems of bronchial congestion, disturbed breathing rhythms, restless-ness, sensitivity to noise, hyperactive behaviour, and fits of depression have all responded to this therapy.

Careful examination of the head will reveal distortions in the symmetry of the cranial bones and disruption of the cranial pulse, which is only detectable by sensitive palpation. The shape of many heads may result from compressive forces during foetal development and others result from stress at birth itself. These seemingly minor trauma are believed by osteopaths to be the cause of interference with the development of the central nervous system, possibly its development during infancy and sometimes its damage at birth. Very early treatment and diagnosis is essential if there is to be any hope of achieving true normal function.

In both children and adults strains on cranial joints can also arise from postural compensation for structural restrictions in other parts of the body, especially the pelvis and foundation of the spine. So also can the reverse apply and strains within the cranium can induce and perpetrate disordered functions in the structures of the rest of the body. These will have all the consequences we have discussed that result from osteopathic lesions. The fascia is very much involved in this connection between the strains within the cranium and those of the rest of the body.

Many difficult persisting conditions which do not always fit medical diagnosis or respond to standard treatment can be greatly assisted by cranial osteopathic techniques. All osteopathic diagnosis seeks to discover how the anatomical characteristics are responsible for disordered function and this is very much the case in cranial diagnosis. Cranial treatment, more than any other, can produce a startling improvement of the symptoms apparently quite unrelated to the refinements of disturbed physical mechanics which interest the osteopath.

A consultation with a cranially trained osteopath can often be very worthwhile both after and before other treatments have been tried.

Chapter 12

Osteopathy in Modern Perspective

How valid are the principles of osteopathy, which were enunciated over one hundred years ago, in the light of modern research and how effective is osteopathic practice when scrutinized in comparison with the results of modern medical treatment?

Osteopathic principles have evolved through experience and increasing enlightenment, and are fundamentally unchanged in spite of many changes in medical therapeutic fashions. As we have seen they are concerned with the body's built-in immunity, with motion, with structure, and function — all of which are matters of natural law.

Both osteopathic and medical research have greatly increased our knowledge in the application of osteopathic principles and confirmed many of the beliefs of the founder. In fact, the more scientific research that is done the more it materially substantiates the idea that structural problems bring about disease-producing processes.

During the last twenty-five years the medical profession has begun to accept the significance of structural problems in conditions such as brachial neuritis, which once was considered to be caused by chemical imbalances in the body. Now physical therapy is the accepted mode of treatment for this and similar disorders. These changes in approach are most noticeable in orthopaedic medicine, where mechanical considerations are necessarily more applicable.

Neurologists, too, have for sometime disregarded the former tendency to think of illness as due purely to defect or disorder in some component of the body and more often they pursue the idea that illness is a vital reaction of the organism as a whole. They consider this reaction to be a response to many adverse factors such as injury, infection, chemical agencies, psychological factors and, not least, nutritional and environmental factors. They point out that all these factors are closely interrelated and they hold the view, for example, that environmental factors can lower people's resistance so that they are more susceptible to infection. Neurologists also take the view that psychological influences such as stress can lead to physical disturbances and eventually cause serious neurological illness.

It would be quite wrong to imply that modern medical practice does not in many areas consider all the influences affecting health, even though in a large majority of cases it appears to be concerned with treating symptoms. Orthodox doctors have, however, been slow to accept the idea that mechanical disorders can also make an individual more susceptible to illness.

Since 1874 there have been immense improvements in the public health service. Medicine has achieved much in the treatment of diseases spread by bacteria and viruses. Diseases previously of major importance, such as syphillis and typhoid, have been displaced from significance by modern therapy. The general practitioner in technically-advanced countries now has a different role. People live longer and as a result suffer from the conditions which accompany old age. Whereas one hundred years ago they were preoccupied with diseases of malnutrition, such as rickets, or with infectious diseases, they now have to cope with osteoarthritis, arthro-sclerosis, high or low blood-pressure, heart problems, etc. The younger patients in general suffer from the neurosis and stress of survival in a technological society. Their complaints are induced by occupational and travelling conditions, over-eating, especially concentrated starch, sugar and protein foods, stuffy ill-ventilated homes, offices and places of entertainment, insufficient exercise and — not least — destructive emotions.

Competitive modern life encourages the pursuit of artificial pleasures, and the need to acquire or experience something new on a regular basis, and much needless worry and exhausting anxiety, is caused by the resulting sense of inadequacy. Stomach ulcers, nervous breakdown and coronary thrombosis are the indentifiable outcomes. All the other causes of stress and constitutional illness we have described, which are related to sedentary and repetitive occupations, faulty posture and osteopathic lesions, are intermixed with these other contributory factors and not only add to but very often help to induce a large number of these conditions. One kind of stress will so lower an individual's resistance that they will become susceptible to illness created by another. A great percentage of illness has become an ecological problem and the average civilized man is not as physically strong as his predecessor by reason of his softer way of life.

Paradoxically these conditions are much more difficult for the physician to treat. Even in times of electronic technology, which has contributed enormously to medical diagnosis, and astounding inventions which can enable researchers actually to witness disease processes taking place, three-quarters of a GP's patients cannot benefit from these achievements.

The differential diagnosis is a complex problem and osteopathy has no more magic means of dealing with illness founded upon stress, the influences of social or working environments, aggressions, or depression than any other alternative. The principles of osteopathy are, however, just as valid when applied to general illness now as they were at the date of their inception — in spite of the radical differences in the causes of the patient's condition.

Dr Still's conception of osteopathic practice was one of *minimum intervention* in disease, that is to say that he only used methods which he considered could help the patients' own natural healing powers to cure themselves. 'Adjuncts are not necessary to the osteopath,' he said.

Osteopathy was to concern itself with health as opposed to disease. It was to be the study of health. Its concern was to find

the very *basic causes* of the *process* which began illness and to
endeavour to alter them — not to intervene in the process or
attempt to suppress it. Symptoms, in Dr Still's view, were a
natural expression of the disease. 'We say *Disease* when we
should say *Effect*. Disease in an abnormal body is just as natural
as is health when all the parts are in order. The fundamental
principles of osteopathy are different from those of any other
system.' He considered disease from a different standpoint, that
it could *result* from 'anatomical abnormalities followed by
physiological discord'. This might have seemed to imply that
osteopathy disagreed with the 'germ theory', which it did not.
The osteopathic contention is that the structurally healthy
individual is less likely to succumb to the dangers of infection
than one with poor posture, osteopathic lesions, or one who is
adversely affected physically by environmental influences or a
victim of poor nutrition. Dr Still also specifically stated that
cases could not be cured when the disease processes had
advanced too far or they had been over-treated with the drugs of
his time.

It has been suggested that Dr Still believed *all* diseases could
be *cured* by osteopathic means. He did not claim this any more
than a modern physician claims that all diseases can be cured by
drug therapy. The fact that he used manual therapy in the
treatment of such conditions as pneumonia may appear bizarre
to those of us who have been brought up to consider that
antibiotics are essential in such illness. But this is a matter of
conditioning and adherence to concepts. Even now manual
therapy is an effective measure when compared with many
alternatives in such disorders. It may be more practical to use
other methods now, and perhaps few are trained or available to
practise manual therapy, but in the majority of cases it would
prove perfectly adequate. It would be illogical if osteopaths
disregarded the advances in medical practice or discoveries
made since Dr Still's time, particularly as it was his ambition to
see practices improved. Osteopaths in the same way as their
orthodox contemporaries, have abandoned practices which
have been superseded by any improved methods more

beneficial for the patient.

The prerequisite in the practice of osteopathy that all basic causes for the illness are, where possible, discovered inevitably leads to the creation of confidence and rapport between the practitioner and patient, which in itself forms part of the treatment. This relationship is infinitely more useful than, say, the administration of a pain-killer without explanation for the pain or the prescription of anti-inflammatory drugs without explanation for the inflammation. If causes are explained, especially if they relate to occupational conditions, developing posture or social habits, there can be no disappointment if no instant relief of symptoms is achieved. The patient understanding the basic underlying causes of the complaint will more readily accept some responsibility for their own health and take part in a programme to reverse its progress.

Dr Still made one very important assertion which is relevant to modern man — that in the physical economy of the individual many systems must work in harmony. The skeleton, the musculature, the fascia, the viscera, the sensory nervous system, the circulatory system etc., involve the whole man. The postural pattern in the human body is a delicate interplay of forces which require perfect control and freedom of mobility of many small parts, not least the joints of the body and, as we have shown, disharmony leads to ill health. *Emotional and mental reactions to the environment more than ever before condition neuromuscular behaviour* and in turn materially affect health.

As civilized human beings our habitual activities are unnatural and consequently create stressful behaviour. When that stress is too great so called 'breakdown' occurs. The mental and physical relationships of our life cannot be separated. Mental and physical fatigue are inextricably connected. Physical stresses may produce anxieties which make us less able to cope with mental stresses. *Restriction of motion* in the structure of the body will induce hypertension in muscles and fatigue in the nerve cells of the body. The whole being is subject to the reaction when such energy is misapplied mentally and physically and the natural rhythm of the body becomes distorted. So the combination of these stresses will bring all the consequences we have outlined; diseases of the organs, chronic illnesses and ultimately irreversible pathological conditions. This process can only be successfully halted by therapies which will have regard to the total psychophysical condition.

A successful osteopath is very busy and builds up mutual respect with his contemporaries in all other disciplines. By treating problems arising from mechanical disorder he will lighten the load of the physician. He will not undermine a patient's confidence in their family doctor but seek to complement their work. The extent to which a patient seeks osteopathic help is very much their own choice. If they simply want to be relieved of acute pains, caused by such things as back disorder, which have not responded to standard treatments all well and good. Should they show an interest in trying to prevent the recurrence of their problem or exploring the possibility of a completely different approach to a distressing illness, they may find that osteopathic methods can work for them both in the short and long term and can bring benefit to many chronic disorders.

Much confusion arises from the commonly-held view that 'osteopathy' is 'joint manipulation'. The type of joint manipulation used by osteopaths is only one of the techniques of osteopathic practice. Regrettably many practitioners of physical therapy claim to be practising osteopathy because they use some kind of manipulation. But however successful they may be they are not practising osteopathy unless they apply osteopathic principles, use an osteopathic approach, and follow osteopathic thinking. This is a very important distinction that cannot be overemphasized.

There is a movement now within the established medical profession which is more willing to tolerate the beliefs of those whose opinions and training differ from their own and some techniques of both osteopathy and acupuncture in particular are being added to medical practice. But sadly those ideas which do not yet fit into their way of thinking are often ignored and considered 'unscientific'. What we have to say about human function should not be restricted only to such facts as can be proved by 'scientific' experiment or we will be forced to omit so much of what is obviously important about the cause of illness. Osteopathic principles, as any other when practised in part, will only succeed in part. The treatment of a broad spectrum of ailments and a vast range of techniques would be neglected if we relied entirely upon laboratory experimental proof.

A non-osteopathic manipulator considers that the purpose of manipulation is to release a joint restriction which he believes is causing the symptoms from which the patient is *currently* suffering. When he releases such restrictions, and the patient consequently feels better, the symptoms and the pain having been relieved, he then assumes that the patient is cured. True osteopathy goes far beyond this precept and appreciates that structural disorders are on the one hand a manifestation of disturbances of the patient's health processes, and on the other hand the pre-disposing and contributing causes of ill health. The osteopath sees his role as a structural mechanic who attempts to alter the progression of those processes of ill health by manual means, so that the patient's own natural resources will be instigated to halt and reverse them.

The same misconception prevails in the use of acupuncture techniques by those who use 'needling' to relieve pain temporarily but ignore the principles of that art, which also has a total concept.

Health now depends upon more variables than it did one hundred years ago and so we realize that no single factor can bring it about; but conscious attention to details borne out by laboratory tests, or relying on instruments, can only simultaneously identify a few of these variables. There is a danger in this that we persuade ourselves that we are attending to some very important issue of health whilst ignoring an infinitude of other factors. In concentrating on details we may miss the obvious.

Chapter 13

Case Histories

The following case histories have been selected to show the range of osteopathic treatment. The references to 'thin type' and 'stocky type' used in these case histories are defined in Chapter 6. They are structural characteristics and not indications of weight.

No histories of patients with 'disc' problems are given as the subject is fully covered in Chapter 9.

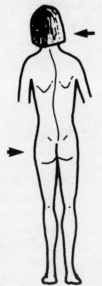

Case History 1

Mary, aged forty-eight was a tall 'thin' type who worked as a shorthand typist. She had a number of basic postural problems. Her left femur was slightly shorter than the right, causing an imbalance in the pelvis which encouraged a curvature of the spine. This was made more pronounced because of the patient's height. Her supporting muscles were long and weak. She carried her head slightly to the left and well forward combining her spinal curvature with a forward stoop. This had been brought about by years of sitting at a typewriter and reading copy from her left hand side.

This patient was suffering from a pain in the left hip with symptoms of numbness in the left leg when typing for a long time. She had pains across her shoulders, headaches and difficulty turning her head to the right when reversing a car. All these symptoms were relieved within one month. Because the patient had longstanding postural problems which were made worse by her occupation no assurance that the symptoms would not return could be given. The patient attended yoga classes and took up regular swimming, with the result that only minor symptoms have occasionally returned.

*   *   *

Case History 2

James, aged fifty-two, was physically well built with good asymmetry and posture. He was a physical worker doing a small amount of lifting and driving a fork lift truck. For four months he had suffered a dull pain in the area of his appendix. His lower abdomen was very sensitive to pressure and there was tension of the muscles and other tissues beneath. Sometimes the patient felt 'lightening'-like pains in the front of his right thigh. After exhaustive medical tests a diagnosis of muscle strain with 'grumbling' appendix was made.

Osteopathic examination showed restriction of the sacrum and lower lumbar vertebrae with some slight shift of the right hip. The patient remembered jumping awkwardly from a trailer five months previously and had slight back pain which did not persist afterwards.

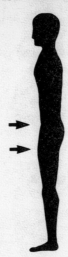

Treatment of the mechanical restrictions relieved all the symptoms within three weeks.

*   *   *

Case History 3
Cathie, aged twenty-seven, was a tall well-built nurse. One year previously she began to experience a very severe pain in her left calf. Her family doctor had prescribed anti-coagulants for six weeks but the pains did not diminish. Blood tests and X-rays had revealed nothing. She subsequently developed an acute burning sensation across her chest and pains on movement of her left shoulder. She was referred to a Consultant Physician who diagnosed fibrositis and rheumatism. An appropriate drug was prescribed but the symptoms persisted and the patient became mentally depressed. Tranquillizers were then prescribed.

This patient had a restriction of her pelvis which had caused referred pains of her leg. Continuing tension from this had disturbed the balance of her posture and induced osteopathic

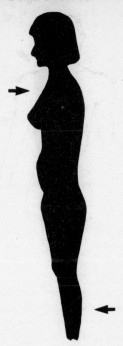

lesions in her upper back which affected her shoulder and chest. Osteopathic treatment was given on the day of consultation, and fourteen days later the patient was much better. She no longer had any pain in her chest or leg although some pain persisted in her shoulder. Three weeks later, after one further treatment, she was completely better both physically and mentally and has had no recurrences of the symptoms since.

* * *

Case History 4
Phillip, aged twenty, had been suffering pains in his left arm for seven months which were worse at night and continual while driving a van which was his chief occupation. Orthopaedic investigation including X-rays of his neck and shoulder had

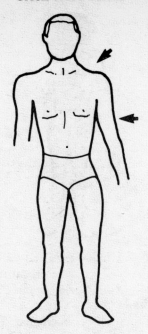

proved negative. Neuritis had been diagnosed. The patient was taking eight painkillers a day.

Osteopathic examination showed a depression of the third rib which was causing his left clavicle to lift. One treatment relieved all the symptoms within three days. The patient recollected suffering pain in his ribs after a Rugby tackle twelve months earlier.

*   *   *

Case History 5
Gwendolen, aged thirty-two, was a petite type with good posture. Four months previously she had suddenly developed pains in her chest while on a coach trip. These pains persisted and spread to the left and were aggravated by bending forward. As she worked in a kindergarten the problem became very

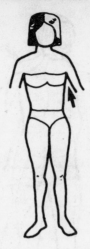

distressing. X-rays and ECG tests requested by her GP had proved negative. She had a barium meal test to eliminate the possibility of the pain being caused by an ulcer. The pain later spread to the left elbow.

Osteopathic examination revealed that she had a restriction of one of her ribs and all the symptoms disappeared after two treatments. She has experienced no pain since.

*   *   *

Case History 6
Janet, aged forty-one, was a 'stocky type' with heavy bone structure. Three years before she had suffered an injury to her lower back in a car accident. She was incapacitated for four months and recovered after a long course of physiotherapy. She had not enjoyed full mobility of her spine since that date and gradually developed a restriction of her right hip. It became necessary for her to support herself with a stick when walking. The strain of walking with this restriction and leaning on this support had caused a compensating change in weight distribution which affected her back higher up and she now suffered headaches and stiffness in the neck.

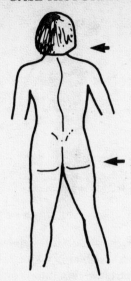

A programme of management involving manipulative treatment and exercises was implemented and the patient was advised to reduce her weight. She conscientiously adhered to both the diet and exercise programme with great determination. Full mobility was restored to her lower back within two months and her headaches and neck stiffness cleared almost immediately. There was gradual improvement in the range of movement of the hip and ultimately fifteen months later she could walk with an easy action and no discomfort. Her previous deportment was restored.

Note: many hip restrictions can be released quickly while others take many months and require the patient to persevere with exercises to achieve success because of the process of alteration and ossification of the inter-articular surfaces. When this is advanced, only surgery can rectify the condition.

*   *   *

Case History 7
Rose, aged forty-one, was employed as an office worker, had a

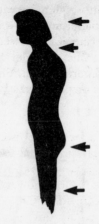

'thin' structure and was of medium height. She had noticeable occupationally induced problems with her posture which were evident on first appearence. For many years she had suffered intermittent attacks of migraine as well as stiffness in her back and shoulders. She took painkillers regularly and had several courses of sedative drugs when problems were particularly distressing. When decorating her house eight months prior to consultation she jolted her back as she stepped from a chair. The next day her low back pain became acute and subsequently worsened progressively. Pains began to radiate down her right leg into her foot. Her family doctor diagnosed sciatica and prescribed strong painkillers. As she was unable to sit for any length of time without severe pain she could not attend her work for seven months.

When examined she was found to have osteopathic lesions in her neck, her upper and lower back. She had a pelvic shift and minor restrictions of her ankles and knees. Full rotation of her hip was not possible. Many of these restrictions of mobility had been present for a long time and were clearly induced by her occupational posture. The final disorganization of her pelvis may very well not have occurred had she enjoyed better overall mobility of her structure. Osteopathic treatment relieved her of the acute sciatic symptoms within three weeks, and she returned to work. Subsequent treatment helped her to overcome her other problems and she was able to give up taking painkillers completely. She was advised to take up yoga and after fourteen months was considerably more flexible and enjoying much better general health. She had no recurrence of migraine or other aches or pains for over one year.

Note

When sciatica is caused by either osteopathic lesions or disc problems it responds well to manual treatment and will nearly always subside within a few weeks of release of the restrictions that bring it about. It is not, however, possible to forecast accurately when pain from the inflamed nerve will stop. In 60 per cent of cases the results are quick but acute pain can sometimes persist after the cause has been removed. Patients can become despondent after having their hopes lifted on initial treatment, but even stubborn symptoms will usually clear within six weeks. Further osteopathic manipulative procedures are not necessary while the patient is awaiting relief but other manual treatments can be of benefit. Sciatica can be caused through strains, which have the effect of stretching the nerve and so inducing inflammation. In these cases no manipulation is necessary and physiotherapy is likely to be more beneficial and suitable. No complete relief from symptoms will ever be obtained in cases where joints are restricted until those restrictions have been released.

*   *   *

Case History 8

Cynthia, aged fifty-two, was a tall slim type. She had a short right leg which, combined with thin muscles and ligaments, had brought about a postural deviation of the neck and head. Four years prior to consultation she had suffered attacks of vertigo and after medical tests Ménières disease had been suspected. She had taken drugs for this condition since that date without any continuing relief of the symptoms. One year before

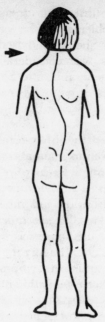

consultation she began to suffer severe pains in the head and neck. She held her head in a very tense way and was frightened to move it freely for fear that the symptoms of disturbed balance should occur. She had treatment every fourteen days for eight weeks and began a programme of very gentle exercises with relaxation techniques.

Fourteen days after the first treatment the pains in her neck had diminished and almost gone. Fourteen days after the third treatment there was a remarkable improvement in her symptoms of imbalance. She had only experienced them once since the previous treatment and the pains had not recurred.

She returned for a check-up two months later and reported only a minor recurrence of imbalance which did not last more than two days. These minor symptoms reappeared in a mild way three months later, since which she has had no further problem. The patient was told to expect some return of the symptoms because of her postural problems and encouraged to keep up ligament stretching exercises indefinitely as a preventative measure.

*   *   *

Case History 9

George, aged fifty-eight, was a tall thin bone type, who since the age of sixteen had worked in a shoe factory. He operated a machine which involved a slow pulling action with his right arm. For many years he had suffered pains in the upper back between the shoulder blades where he developed a curvature (occupational hump). During the winter of 1982 he was taken ill with nausea, vomiting and diarrhoea. His family doctor prescribed rest and later anti-nauseants when the symptoms did not subside after a week. All the acute symptoms then stopped but the patient continued to experience 'shivers', developed a sharp pain in the costal arch and mid back as well as generally becoming depressed. Hospital investigation revealed no causes for the symptoms and after examination by a Consultant a diagnosis of suspected pancreatitis was made. Four months

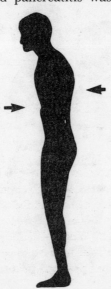

later the patient was still unable to attend work because of pain, depression and involuntary 'shivering'. Osteopathic examination in September 1983 revealed a restriction of the eighth thoracic vertebra and restriction of the ribs attached to it. Release of this lesion and relaxation of the diaphragm resulted in a spectacular relief of pain. Further manual treatment given in the area of the upper abdomen with general osteopathic management over a period of three months coincided with the gradual diminution of the symptoms. The patient was advised to request his employer to give him a different job so as not to continually strain his thorax and shoulders.

*   *   *

Case Histories 10 and 11

Jean and Gillian aged fifty-seven and fifty-nine respectively, were sisters. They had both been shoe operatives all their working lives. They were both 'thin' types of medium height. Both had developed pains in the shoulder and neck and right

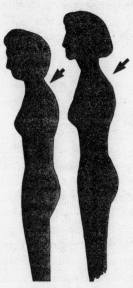

arm within a period of eighteen months. They both had pins and needles in the fingers and some headaches. Jean had been referred to a specialist for consultation who recommended a carpal tunnel operation (an incision into the wrist to divide the ligaments and the bones beneath, thereby permitting improvement of circulation to the hands).

Osteopathic examination revealed that both sisters had altered posture in the lower back and pelvis, round shoulders and slight side carriage of the head arising from the position in which they each sat at work. They both had restrictions of the joints immediately below the neck and in the lower back. They had some wear on their joints but no evidence of advanced arthritis. Osteopathic treatment brought complete relief of all the symptoms from which Jean was suffering within six weeks and operation was unnecessary. Her sister Gillian was relieved of the pains in her shoulders, neck and arm, but the pins and needles in her hand continued. After two months she was recommended to ask her GP to refer her to a Consultant and six months later she underwent a carpal tunnel operation and the residual symptoms were relieved. Both sisters were advised to use a simple exercise routine to keep their necks and shoulders as mobile as possible and compensate for the long hours of working in static positions.

*   *   *

Case History 12

Geoffrey, aged twenty-six was a lorry driver. A well-built, medium height 'thin' type, for six months he had continually experienced stabbing pains in the lower part of his chest which later radiated upwards. X-rays and ECG tests had been negative. The patient was taking painkillers while continuing work.

Examination showed that he had restrictions in the mid-spinal joints which were confining the movement of his diaphragm. The areas of the gall bladder and stomach were painful when examined. Osteopathic treatment was given to

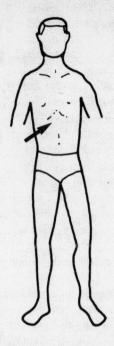

release his spinal restrictions and the gall bladder was manually drained. The patient was relieved of the symptoms within a week. He has reported no problems since.

* * *

Case History 13

Edward, aged fifty-two, was an office worker. An upright 'thin' type with some sagging of the abdomen caused through lack of physical activity and constant sitting at a desk. For five months he had suffered from an unsubduable need to void the bladder frequently along with pressure while doing so and was receiving drug therapy for this. While gardening he pulled his lower back muscles and consequently suffered a pounding pain in the kidney area.

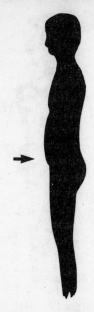

Osteopathic examination revealed restriction of the second lumbar vertebra and also pelvic strain. Adjustment of these relieved the pains. Manual release of adhesions in the abdominal/bladder area quickly relieved the patient of his urinary problems. He returned for treatment two months later after a less severe spell and has since enjoyed normal habits. He now attends a gymnasium for regular light exercises to improve the tone of his abdominal muscles.

*   *   *

Case History 14

Neil, aged sixty, was a stocky type with no evidence of postural problems. He was slightly overweight and had a physical occupation. He had suffered severe pains in the left side of his chest for three months which were worse at night and so interfering with his sleep. Full medical investigation had confirmed no 'heart disorder' and the possibility of stomach

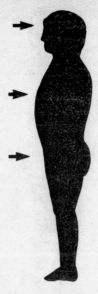

problems had been eliminated. The patient was prescribed sleeping pills and painkillers to be taken when needed only. Possible strain of the muscles around the rib cage was diagnosed. The patient then began to experience malaise and was apt to feel dizzy. He also felt the need to void his bladder more frequently.

Osteopathic examination revealed restrictions of the sixth thoracic vertebra and some restriction of movement of the left shoulder as well as tightness in the lower neck. Treatment relieved the symptoms of pain within two weeks. The patient was then able to give up taking sleeping pills and normal sleep was restored. Other attendant symptoms disappeared within a month.

*   *   *

Case History 15
Vera, aged forty-two, came for treatment because she had read in a magazine that osteopathic treatment could sometimes help

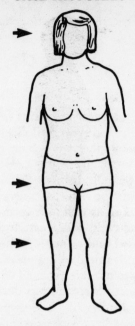

insomnia. She was a stocky type and overweight. She had until one year previously always been 'a good sleeper'. She now found that she was waking up about 3 a.m. every morning and not sleeping again until about 7 a.m. when it was almost time to get up. She had no domestic or financial problems and no history of nervous disorder or stress.

Consultation brought to light that she had suffered dyspepsia for over eighteen months and felt a fullness around her heart especially during the evenings. Also she had suffered dysmenorrhoea ten months previously which had been relieved with medication but returned in a mild way since. Very considerable muscle tension and restriction was found in this patient's shoulder girdle with minor osteopathic lesions. By relaxing this and the whole thoracic area several times during a period of two months the patient began to regain her normal sleeping habits. Osteopathic treatment of the back, pelvis and abdomen was followed by complete relief of all her remaining symptoms. She was recommended to reduce weight and take regular exercise.

*   *   *

Case History 16

Malcolm, aged four, had suffered pains in both heels for over two years. Usually the pains were dull and at a low level of registration. Occasionally they were sharp and sudden, causing the child to cry out, especially at night. His playgroup teacher had reported him to be dull, disinterested and mildly unhappy.

Osteopathic examination detected a very minor restriction of the fifth lumbar vertebra as well as a vertical strain at the very top of his spine. The child was treated once a week for two months. Very modified and minor movement was introduced into his lower back and cranial techniques were used to treat the head area. The symptoms were relieved within one month and have not returned since. Malcolm has developed into an alert leader at infant school.

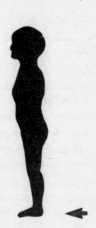

Where to Find Your Osteopath

As there is no state registration of osteopaths in the UK general medical practitioners exercise caution when referring patients to them. A good osteopath's reputation will be his reference, especially in a provincial area. Family doctors will usually pass the names of those established osteopaths who from experience they have learned to trust. Any patient may consult an osteopath without being referred by a GP.

The reputable colleges of osteopathy keep registers of all practising members who have qualified from their institutions as well as those who they consider hold other satisfactory qualifications. Prospective patients who have not been referred to an osteopath may obtain full registers of qualified practitioners from the addresses below. Some registers are available in public libraries. When making an appointment patients should indicate the kind of problem they have so that the practitioner may decide whether he is able to help the particular condition.

British College of Naturopathy
  and Osteopathy
Frazer House
6 Netherhall Gardens
London NW3 5RR.
Tel. 01-435 7830

British School of Osteopathy
1–4 Suffolk Street
London SW1Y 4HG.
Tel. 01-839 2060

The College of Osteopaths
Administrative Services
110 Thorkhill Road
Thames Ditton
Surrey KT7 0UW.
Tel. 01-398 3308

European School of Osteopathy
104 Tonbridge Road
Maidstone
Kent ME16 8SL.
Tel. (0622) 671558

Cranial Osteopathic Association
  (UK)
478 Baker St
Enfield
Middlesex EN1 3QS

American Osteopathic Association
and Canadian Osteopathic
  Association
P.O. Bin 1050
Carmel
California 93921
USA

Australia Osteopathic Association
71 Collins Street
Victoria
Australia

Holistic Medical Centre
1412 North Broadway
Lexington
Kentucky 40505
USA

American Academy of
  Osteopathy
(Business Office)
2630 Airport Road
Colorado Springs
Colorado 80910
USA

New Zealand Register of
  Osteopaths
92 Hurstmere Road
Takapuna
Auckland 9
New Zealand

Index

In the same series...

ACUPUNCTURE

A Patient's Guide

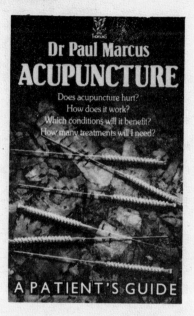

Dr Paul Marcus. A complete practical guide for the patient contemplating treatment by acupuncture. Uses western scientific explanations to describe acupuncture therapy in all its aspects in language a lay reader can easily understand. Dr Marcus, a medically trained practising acupuncturist, explains what a patient can expect from acupuncture and answers such questions as: Does acupuncture hurt? How does it work? What are the dangers? With an account of the history of acupuncture and a simple explanation of the facts so far known, it provides a refreshingly modern approach to a subject we all should know about. Contents include: which illnesses respond to acupuncture: how treatment is carried out; treatment with needles and moxibustion; the disadvantages and case histories.